Personalized Medicine for Orthopaedic Disorders

Personalized Medicine for Orthopaedic Disorders

Editor

Nan Jiang

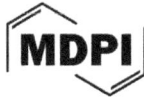

Basel • Beijing • Wuhan • Barcelona • Belgrade • Novi Sad • Cluj • Manchester

Editor
Nan Jiang
Southern Medical University
Nanfang Hospital
Guangzhou
China

Editorial Office
MDPI
St. Alban-Anlage 66
4052 Basel, Switzerland

This is a reprint of articles from the Special Issue published online in the open access journal *Journal of Personalized Medicine* (ISSN 2075-4426) (available at: https://www.mdpi.com/journal/jpm/special_issues/3R4169ZJ0K).

For citation purposes, cite each article independently as indicated on the article page online and as indicated below:

Lastname, A.A.; Lastname, B.B. Article Title. *Journal Name* **Year**, *Volume Number*, Page Range.

ISBN 978-3-7258-1057-4 (Hbk)
ISBN 978-3-7258-1058-1 (PDF)
doi.org/10.3390/books978-3-7258-1058-1

© 2024 by the authors. Articles in this book are Open Access and distributed under the Creative Commons Attribution (CC BY) license. The book as a whole is distributed by MDPI under the terms and conditions of the Creative Commons Attribution-NonCommercial-NoDerivs (CC BY-NC-ND) license.

Contents

About the Editor vii

Nan Jiang
Personalized Medicine for Orthopaedic Disorders
Reprinted from: *J. Pers. Med.* **2023**, *13*, 1553, doi:10.3390/jpm13111553 1

Wanrun Zhong, Yanmao Wang, Hongshu Wang, Pei Han, Yi Sun, Yimin Chai, et al.
Bacterial Contamination of Open Fractures: Pathogens and Antibiotic Resistance Patterns in East China
Reprinted from: *J. Pers. Med.* **2023**, *13*, 735, doi:10.3390/jpm13050735 4

Yang Yu, Qunshan Lu, Songlin Li, Mingxing Liu, Houyi Sun, Lei Li, et al.
Intra-Articular Injection of Autologous Micro-Fragmented Adipose Tissue for the Treatment of Knee Osteoarthritis: A Prospective Interventional Study
Reprinted from: *J. Pers. Med.* **2023**, *13*, 504, doi:10.3390/jpm13030504 13

Jintao Xu, Kai Chen, Yaohui Yu, Yishu Wang, Yi Zhu, Xiangjie Zou and Yiqiu Jiang
Identification of Immune-Related Risk Genes in Osteoarthritis Based on Bioinformatics Analysis and Machine Learning
Reprinted from: *J. Pers. Med.* **2023**, *13*, 367, doi:10.3390/jpm13020367 25

Matthew A. Wysocki and Scott T. Doyle
Advancing Osteoporosis Evaluation Procedures: Detailed Computational Analysis of Regional Structural Vulnerabilities in Osteoporotic Bone
Reprinted from: *J. Pers. Med.* **2023**, *13*, 321, doi:10.3390/jpm13020321 38

Vilim Molnar, Eduard Pavelić, Željko Jeleč, Petar Brlek, Vid Matišić, Igor Borić, et al.
Results of Treating Mild to Moderate Knee Osteoarthritis with Autologous Conditioned Adipose Tissue and Leukocyte-Poor Platelet-Rich Plasma
Reprinted from: *J. Pers. Med.* **2022**, *13*, 47, doi:10.3390/jpm13010047 53

Peng Chen, Qing-rong Lin, Mou-Zhang Huang, Xin Zhang, Yan-jun Hu, Jing Chen, et al.
Devascularized Bone Surface Culture: A Novel Strategy for Identifying Osteomyelitis-Related Pathogens
Reprinted from: *J. Pers. Med.* **2022**, *12*, 2050, doi:10.3390/jpm12122050 68

Weiran Hu, Guang Yang, Hongqiang Wang, Xiaonan Wu, Haohao Ma, Kai Zhang and Yanzheng Gao
Which Is Better in Clinical and Radiological Outcomes for Lumbar Degenerative Disease of Two Segments: MIS-TLIF or OPEN-TLIF?
Reprinted from: *J. Pers. Med.* **2022**, *12*, 1977, doi:10.3390/jpm12121977 79

Chris Lindemann, Timo Zippelius, Felix Hochberger, Alexander Hölzl, Sabrina Böhle and Patrick Strube
Local Infiltrations in Patients with Radiculopathy or Chronic Low Back Pain Due to Segment Degeneration—Only A Diagnostic Value?
Reprinted from: *J. Pers. Med.* **2022**, *12*, 1791, doi:10.3390/jpm12111791 89

Cristina Molina-García, Andrés Reinoso-Cobo, Jonathan Cortés-Martín, Eva Lopezosa-Reca, Ana Marchena-Rodriguez, George Banwell and Laura Ramos-Petersen
Efficacy of Personalized Foot Orthoses in Children with Flexible Flat Foot: Protocol for a Randomized Controlled Trial
Reprinted from: *J. Pers. Med.* **2023**, *13*, 1269, doi:10.3390/jpm13081269 101

Davide Maria Maggioni, Riccardo Giorgino, Carmelo Messina, Domenico Albano, Giuseppe Michele Peretti and Laura Mangiavini
Framing Patellar Instability: From Diagnosis to the Treatment of the First Episode
Reprinted from: *J. Pers. Med.* **2023**, *13*, 1225, doi:10.3390/jpm13081225 . . . . **115**

René Schwesig, George Fieseler, Jakob Cornelius, Julia Sendler, Stephan Schulze, Souhail Hermassi, et al.
A Longitudinal Analysis of the Internal Rotation and Shift (IRO/Shift) Test Following Arthroscopic Repair of Superior Rotator Cuff Lesions
Reprinted from: *J. Pers. Med.* **2022**, *12*, 2018, doi:10.3390/jpm12122018 . . . . **127**

About the Editor

Nan Jiang

Nan Jiang is an orthopedic surgeon at the Southern Medical University Nanfang Hospital in Guangzhou, China. He obtained his MD from the Southern Medical University, China, in 2016. His primary research interests revolve around fracture-related infections and evidence-based Orthopedics and Traumatology. He is an active member of the European Bone and Joint Infection Society (EBJIS) and the International Chinese Musculoskeletal Research Society (ICMRS). In 2019, he was a visiting scholar, researching bacterial biofilms at Dr. Paul Stoodley's lab within the Department of Microbial Infection and Immunity, Wexner Medical Center, Ohio State University, OH, USA. He serves as an editorial member for the International Journal of Immunogenetics and BMC Musculoskeletal Disorders. In 2023, he was appointed as an Associate Researcher in Orthopedics.

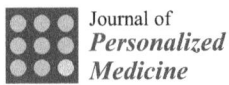

Editorial

Personalized Medicine for Orthopaedic Disorders

Nan Jiang

Division of Orthopaedics & Traumatology, Department of Orthopaedics, Nanfang Hospital, Southern Medical University, Guangzhou 510515, China; hnxyjn@smu.edu.cn

Orthopaedic disorders, also known as musculoskeletal disorders (MSDs), refer to diseases or injuries of the bone, joint, cartilage, muscle, tendon, nerve, and spinal disc. As MSDs display characteristics of complexity and high heterogeneity, clinical diagnosis is sometimes difficult and treatment is often tricky. Take osteomyelitis as an example, which presently still poses great challenges to orthopaedic surgeons while clinical efficacy remains unsatisfactory. Meanwhile, such a disorder aggravates the economic burden of the patients and their families. According to a recent survey, the median healthcare cost of patients with post-traumatic osteomyelitis was almost five-fold higher than that for those without infection [1]. In addition, patients with osteomyelitis experienced high risks of comorbidity, such as epilepsy [2], diabetes mellitus [3], and even depression [4]. These suggest great influences of osteomyelitis on the patients, both physically and psychologically.

In order to keep up with the latest knowledge in the fields of MSDs, this Special Issue was set up with the aim of collecting current investigations focusing on MSDs. In total, we received twenty-three submissions and after evaluations by the editorial office staff, myself, and the peer reviewers, and we finally accepted eleven papers, including six articles, two communications, two study protocols and one perspective. Here, I briefly introduce the eleven articles in this Special Issue.

In a prospective study, Lindemann et al. [5] investigated the therapeutic effectiveness of CT-assisted infiltration with respect to pain, function, and life quality between two different kinds of injections (periradicular infiltration, PRI versus facet joint capsule infiltration, FJI) in chronic complaints. The outcomes of 87 patients from FJI group and 109 patients from PRI group demonstrated that PRI, not FJI, is an easy and suitable strategy to provide a durable therapeutic value for patients with chronic radicular pain and related low back pain.

In a retrospective study, Hu et al. [6] compared the efficacy between minimally invasive transforaminal lumbar interbody fusion (MIS-TLIF) and traditional open transforaminal lumbar interbody fusion (OPEN-TLIF) for the management of two-level lumbar degenerative disorders. Outcomes revealed that similar results were obtained regarding the life quality after surgery, radiological findings, risks of muscle injury and other types of complications between the two groups. However, patients that received MIS-TLIF had a longer surgical time and more radiation exposures during surgery than those by OPEN-TLIF. In addition, patients in the MIS-TLIF group also experienced a higher risk regarding the pedicle screws deviating laterally out of the vertebral body. Thus, they recommended the OPEN-TLIF technique for the treatment of two-level lumbar degenerative diseases.

In a prospective, blinded study, Schwesig et al. [7] compared the accuracy of the internal rotation and Shift (IRO/Shift) test with the Jobe test for evaluation of the recovery following arthroscopic repair of the superior rotator cuff at 3 and 6 months after surgery. Based on the outcomes of the 51 patients included, the authors concluded that the accuracy of the IRO/Shift test was better than the Jobe test, though the accuracy of both tests improved between 3 and 6 months after surgery.

In a prospective study, Chen et al. [8] introduced a novel method, named devascularized bone surface culture (BSC), with comparison to the traditional tissue sampling culture (TSC),

Citation: Jiang, N. Personalized Medicine for Orthopaedic Disorders. *J. Pers. Med.* **2023**, *13*, 1553. https://doi.org/10.3390/jpm13111553

Received: 17 October 2023
Accepted: 22 October 2023
Published: 30 October 2023

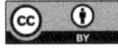

Copyright: © 2023 by the author. Licensee MDPI, Basel, Switzerland. This article is an open access article distributed under the terms and conditions of the Creative Commons Attribution (CC BY) license (https:// creativecommons.org/licenses/by/ 4.0/).

for identifying osteomyelitis-related microorganisms. According to the results of 51 patients, the authors reported that the detectable rate following BSC was relatively higher than that of the TSC (75% vs. 59%, $p = 0.093$). Meanwhile, the median culture time following BSC was significantly shorter than the TSC (1 day vs. 3 days, $p < 0.001$). Therefore, they concluded that BSC may be better than TSC for detecting osteomyelitis-related microorganisms.

In a prospective, non-randomized, interventional trial, Molnar et al. [9] assessed clinical efficacy following the use of autologous conditioned adipose tissue (ACA) and leukocyte-poor PRP (LP-PRP) in patients with mild to moderate knee osteoarthritis (KOA). The outcomes of 16 patients revealed that the combination of ACA and LP-PRP, as a minimally invasive approach, offered excellent improvements in symptoms among the patients with mild to moderate KOA.

In a cadaveric and computational-analysis-based study, Wysocki et al. [10] examined the differences of femoral structures and geometric properties between healthy and osteoporotic bones. The outcomes of 42 cadaveric CT data showed that statistical differences were found regarding multiple geometric properties between healthy and osteoporotic femoral bones. Such differences of the geometric properties are evident locally. In addition, this study also demonstrated the feasibility of using CT-scans-based 3D models for analysing the differences in femoral shapes and related biomechanical properties.

In a bioinformatics analysis- and machine-learning-based study, Xu et al. [11] conducted a bioinformatic analysis of immune cell infiltration in cartilage and synovium of OA, and identified three potential risk genes, *PTGS1*, *HLA-DMB* and *GPR137B*. These genes were found to interact with the immune system in OA, which provides a feasible direction for future drug research and development for this disorder.

In a prospective interventional study, Yu et al. [12] assessed the efficacy and safety of using autologous micro-fragmented adipose tissue (MF-AT) for improving joint function and repairing cartilage in KOA patients. Based on the outcomes of 20 patients, the authors concluded that autologous MF-AT can help improve the knee function and relieve pain without adverse events. Nonetheless, the improved knee function failed to be sustained, with the best results occurring at 9 to 12 months after intervention and the cartilage regeneration still needing to be further explored.

In a retrospective multicentre study conducted in six healthcare centres in Eastern China, Zhong et al. [13] characterized the bacterial spectrum following open fractures and analysed the situations of bacterial resistance to antibiotics from 2015 to 2017. The data of 1348 patients showed that the positive rate of culture following open fractures was about 55%, 59% of which were detected in grade III fractures. It was noted that approximate 73% of the identified pathogens were sensitive to prophylactic antibiotics, with quinolones and cotrimoxazole showing the lowest resistant rates. Based on the findings, the authors suggested supplemental antibiotics to cover for Gram-negative bacteria for grade II open fractures.

In a perspective study, Maggioni et al. [14] systematically introduced patellar instability, including the classification of patellofemoral disorders, principal factors of instability, patellofemoral instability, diagnosis, treatment options and follow-up for primary dislocation. This can help readers better understand the clinical diagnosis and treatment of patellar instability.

In a protocol of a randomized controlled trial (RCT), Molina-García et al. [15] focused on the clinical efficacy of foot orthoses (FO) for the treatment of paediatric flat foot (PFF). Through this RCT, they aimed to determine if personalized FO, combined with a specific exercise regimen, could produce results similar to or even better than only specific exercises. The authors hypothesized that such a combination can better improve the signs and symptoms of PFF.

In summary, the studies included in this Special Issue cover different areas regarding epidemiology, diagnosis, and treatment of different types of MSDs. In the future, more investigations with high-level evidence are required to drive our progress toward improving our knowledge to meet the challenges and future prospects of MSDs.

Funding: This research received no external funding.

Acknowledgments: I would like to thank all the authors who submitted their excellent work to this Special Issue. Moreover, I am also very grateful to the *Journal of Personalized Medicine* for providing me the opportunity to be the Guest Editor of this Special Issue, and in particular, I would like to thank the working staff of the journal for their great help.

Conflicts of Interest: The author declares no conflict of interest.

References

1. Jiang, N.; Wu, H.T.; Lin, Q.R.; Hu, Y.J.; Yu, B. Health Care Costs of Post-traumatic Osteomyelitis in China: Current Situation and Influencing Factors. *J. Surg. Res.* **2020**, *247*, 356–363. [CrossRef] [PubMed]
2. Tseng, C.H.; Huang, W.S.; Muo, C.H.; Kao, C.H. Increased risk of epilepsy among patients diagnosed with chronic osteomyelitis. *Epilepsy Res* **2014**, *108*, 1427–1434. [CrossRef] [PubMed]
3. Lin, S.Y.; Lin, C.L.; Tseng, C.H.; Wang, I.K.; Wang, S.M.; Huang, C.C.; Chang, Y.J.; Kao, C.H. The association between chronic osteomyelitis and increased risk of diabetes mellitus: A population-based cohort study. *Eur. J. Clin. Microbiol. Infect. Dis. Off. Publ. Eur. Soc. Clin. Microbiol.* **2014**, *33*, 1647–1652. [CrossRef] [PubMed]
4. Tseng, C.H.; Huang, W.S.; Muo, C.H.; Chang, Y.J.; Kao, C.H. Increased depression risk among patients with chronic osteomyelitis. *J. Psychosom. Res.* **2014**, *77*, 535–540. [CrossRef] [PubMed]
5. Lindemann, C.; Zippelius, T.; Hochberger, F.; Holzl, A.; Bohle, S.; Strube, P. Local Infiltrations in Patients with Radiculopathy or Chronic Low Back Pain Due to Segment Degeneration-Only A Diagnostic Value? *J. Pers. Med.* **2022**, *12*, 1791. [CrossRef] [PubMed]
6. Hu, W.; Yang, G.; Wang, H.; Wu, X.; Ma, H.; Zhang, K.; Gao, Y. Which Is Better in Clinical and Radiological Outcomes for Lumbar Degenerative Disease of Two Segments: MIS-TLIF or OPEN-TLIF? *J. Pers. Med.* **2022**, *12*, 1977. [CrossRef] [PubMed]
7. Schwesig, R.; Fieseler, G.; Cornelius, J.; Sendler, J.; Schulze, S.; Hermassi, S.; Delank, K.S.; Laudner, K. A Longitudinal Analysis of the Internal Rotation and Shift (IRO/Shift) Test Following Arthroscopic Repair of Superior Rotator Cuff Lesions. *J. Pers. Med.* **2022**, *12*, 2018. [CrossRef] [PubMed]
8. Chen, P.; Lin, Q.R.; Huang, M.Z.; Zhang, X.; Hu, Y.J.; Chen, J.; Jiang, N.; Yu, B. Devascularized Bone Surface Culture: A Novel Strategy for Identifying Osteomyelitis-Related Pathogens. *J. Pers. Med.* **2022**, *12*, 2050. [CrossRef] [PubMed]
9. Molnar, V.; Pavelic, E.; Jelec, Z.; Brlek, P.; Matisic, V.; Boric, I.; Hudetz, D.; Rod, E.; Vidovic, D.; Starcevic, N.; et al. Results of Treating Mild to Moderate Knee Osteoarthritis with Autologous Conditioned Adipose Tissue and Leukocyte-Poor Platelet-Rich Plasma. *J. Pers. Med.* **2022**, *13*, 47. [CrossRef] [PubMed]
10. Wysocki, M.A.; Doyle, S.T. Advancing Osteoporosis Evaluation Procedures: Detailed Computational Analysis of Regional Structural Vulnerabilities in Osteoporotic Bone. *J. Pers. Med.* **2023**, *13*, 321. [CrossRef] [PubMed]
11. Xu, J.; Chen, K.; Yu, Y.; Wang, Y.; Zhu, Y.; Zou, X.; Jiang, Y. Identification of Immune-Related Risk Genes in Osteoarthritis Based on Bioinformatics Analysis and Machine Learning. *J. Pers. Med.* **2023**, *13*, 367. [CrossRef] [PubMed]
12. Yu, Y.; Lu, Q.; Li, S.; Liu, M.; Sun, H.; Li, L.; Han, K.; Liu, P. Intra-Articular Injection of Autologous Micro-Fragmented Adipose Tissue for the Treatment of Knee Osteoarthritis: A Prospective Interventional Study. *J. Pers. Med.* **2023**, *13*, 504. [CrossRef] [PubMed]
13. Zhong, W.; Wang, Y.; Wang, H.; Han, P.; Sun, Y.; Chai, Y.; Lu, S.; Hu, C. Bacterial Contamination of Open Fractures: Pathogens and Antibiotic Resistance Patterns in East China. *J. Pers. Med.* **2023**, *13*, 735. [CrossRef] [PubMed]
14. Maggioni, D.M.; Giorgino, R.; Messina, C.; Albano, D.; Peretti, G.M.; Mangiavini, L. Framing Patellar Instability: From Diagnosis to the Treatment of the First Episode. *J. Pers. Med.* **2023**, *13*, 1225. [CrossRef] [PubMed]
15. Molina-Garcia, C.; Reinoso-Cobo, A.; Cortes-Martin, J.; Lopezosa-Reca, E.; Marchena-Rodriguez, A.; Banwell, G.; Ramos-Petersen, L. Efficacy of Personalized Foot Orthoses in Children with Flexible Flat Foot: Protocol for a Randomized Controlled Trial. *J. Pers. Med.* **2023**, *13*, 1269. [CrossRef]

Disclaimer/Publisher's Note: The statements, opinions and data contained in all publications are solely those of the individual author(s) and contributor(s) and not of MDPI and/or the editor(s). MDPI and/or the editor(s) disclaim responsibility for any injury to people or property resulting from any ideas, methods, instructions or products referred to in the content.

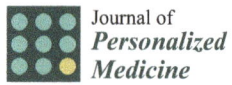

Communication

Bacterial Contamination of Open Fractures: Pathogens and Antibiotic Resistance Patterns in East China

Wanrun Zhong †, Yanmao Wang †, Hongshu Wang, Pei Han, Yi Sun, Yimin Chai, Shengdi Lu and Chengfang Hu *

Department of Orthopaedics, Shanghai Sixth People's Hospital Affiliated to Shanghai Jiao Tong University School of Medicine, Shanghai 200235, China; lushendi0828@163.com (S.L.)
* Correspondence: cfhu6thhosp@163.com
† These authors contributed equally to this work.

Abstract: Bacterial contamination of soft tissue in open fractures leads to high infection rates. Pathogens and their resistance against therapeutic agents change with time and vary in different regions. The purpose of this study was to characterize the bacterial spectrum present in open fractures and analyze the bacterial resistance to antibiotic agents based on five trauma centers in East China. A retrospective multicenter cohort study was conducted in six major trauma centers in East China from January 2015 to December 2017. Patients who sustained open fractures of the lower extremities were included. The data collected included the mechanism of injury, the Gustilo-Anderson classification, the isolated pathogens and their resistance against therapeutic agents, as well as the prophylactic antibiotics administered. In total, 1348 patients were included in our study, all of whom received antibiotic prophylaxis (cefotiam or cefuroxime) during the first debridement at the emergency room. Wound cultures were taken in 1187 patients (85.8%); the results showed that the positive rate of open fracture was 54.8% (651/1187), and 59% of the bacterial detections occurred in grade III fractures. Most pathogens (72.7%) were sensitive to prophylactic antibiotics, according to the EAST guideline. Quinolones and cotrimoxazole showed the lowest rates of resistance. The updated EAST guidelines for antibiotic prophylaxis in open fracture (2011) have been proven to be adequate for a large portion of patients, and we would like to suggest additional Gram-negative coverage for patients with grade II open fractures based on the results obtained in this setting in East China.

Keywords: bacterial contamination; open fractures; pathogens; East China

1. Introduction

The frequency of open fractures observed in any area varies according to geographical and socioeconomic factors, population size, and the system of trauma care. Open fractures are common in East China due to the rapid development of the manufacturing and transportation industries. As the infection rates of soft tissues and bones resulting from bacterial contamination have increased up to 50% [1], the incidence of complications, such as acute or delayed osteomyelitis, nonunion, or secondary amputation, may also increase. Although the factors contributing to infection after open fractures vary from person to person, infection prevention measures, including radical debridement and antibiotic prophylaxis, remain critical.

The current options for treating drug-resistant bacteria and bacterial infections include:

(1) Antibiotics: Antibiotics are the most common treatment for bacterial infections. They work by killing or stopping the growth of bacteria. However, some bacteria have become resistant to antibiotics, making it difficult to treat the infections caused by these bacteria. In some cases, stronger antibiotics may be used to treat drug-resistant infections.

(2) Combination therapy: Combination therapy involves using two or more antibiotics together to treat an infection. This can be helpful in treating drug-resistant bacteria, as it may be more effective than using a single antibiotic.

Citation: Zhong, W.; Wang, Y.; Wang, H.; Han, P.; Sun, Y.; Chai, Y.; Lu, S.; Hu, C. Bacterial Contamination of Open Fractures: Pathogens and Antibiotic Resistance Patterns in East China. *J. Pers. Med.* **2023**, *13*, 735. https://doi.org/10.3390/jpm13050735

Academic Editors: Norio Yamamoto and Weikuan Gu

Received: 11 January 2023
Revised: 23 April 2023
Accepted: 24 April 2023
Published: 26 April 2023

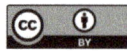

Copyright: © 2023 by the authors. Licensee MDPI, Basel, Switzerland. This article is an open access article distributed under the terms and conditions of the Creative Commons Attribution (CC BY) license (https://creativecommons.org/licenses/by/4.0/).

(3) Probiotics: Probiotics are live bacteria and yeasts that are beneficial to the body. They can help restore the natural balance of bacteria in the gut, which can be disrupted by antibiotics. Probiotics can also boost the immune system and help fight off infections.

(4) Antimicrobial stewardship: Antimicrobial stewardship is a coordinated effort to optimize the use of antibiotics and other antimicrobial drugs. This can involve educating healthcare providers on appropriate prescribing practices, monitoring the use of antibiotics, and implementing guidelines for the use of antibiotics in specific clinical situations.

The Eastern Association for the Surgery of Trauma (EAST) Practice Management Guidelines for prophylactic antibiotic use in open fractures were mainly based on literature emanating from the USA, Canada, Australia, Israel, South Africa, Ethiopia, and Saudi Arabia. No Asian studies were taken into consideration. However, pathogens and their resistance against antibiotic agents change with time and vary in different regions [2–4].

In this study, we aimed to characterize the bacterial spectrum present in open fractures, analyze the bacterial resistance to antibiotic agents, and examine the therapeutic regimes in trauma centers in East China.

2. Materials and Methods

The study protocol was approved by the Ethics Committee of the Shanghai Jiao Tong University Affiliated Sixth People's Hospital. Informed consent was obtained from all participants. All study methods were in accordance with the Declaration of Helsinki.

The pathogens and antibiotic resistance patterns of open fractures in East China were analyzed using data collected as part of a multicenter study (an epidemiological investigation of traumatic infections of the upper and lower extremities) that was designed to analyze the pathogens, antibiotic resistance patterns, and risk factors for soft tissue and/or bone infection after an open fracture.

Six trauma centers in East China participated in this retrospective and prospective cohort study. Patients' data from six of the seven states in East China were covered in this multicenter study.

The study protocol was approved by the institutional review boards of each of the centers. All of the patients consented to participate in the study, including follow-up evaluations.

We included all patients who sustained open fractures from January 2015 to December 2017 at six trauma centers. The patients' data, as well as their Gustilo-Anderson classification, were noted, and the data were collected anonymously at the participating trauma centers with an Excel form and transferred to an SPSS chart. Bacterial contamination was assessed using deep tissue samples, and antibiotic resistance patterns were assessed using VITEK®® 2 (BioMérieux, Marcy-l'Étoile, France).

3. Results

Each of the six centers included in this study was the largest trauma center in the state where it was located. In total, 1348 patients were included, with ages ranging from 16 to 82 years, with a mean of 37.5 years. Eight hundred and eighty-seven patients were male (64.1%).

The etiologies were mostly road traffic accidents (1107 patients, 80.0%). The lower leg (728 patients, 52.6%) and hand (519 patients, 37.5%) were the most commonly injured locations in this study. Most patients in this study had Gustilo-Anderson grade II open fractures (578 patients, 42.9%).

All patients received prophylactic antibiotics during the first debridement at the emergency room (Table 1). Microbiological samples were taken from the deep tissues of the fracture site in 545 patients (40.4%). Swabs taken from the wounds were cultivated in 339 patients (25.1%), and tissue samples were taken from 103 patients (7.6%). Most of the samples (558 samples, 56.5%) were drawn from patients with Gustilo-Anderson grade II open fractures. Intraoperative samples, or swabs, were collected from all patients who sustained Gustilo-Anderson grade III open fractures.

Table 1. Prophylactic antibiotics according to the Gustilo-Anderson classification.

Gustilo-Anderson Classification	Prophylactic Antibiotics	n
I	Cefazolin	114 (30.6%)
	Cefuroxime	240 (64.3%)
	Clindamycin	19 (5.1%)
II	Cefazolin	187 (32.4%)
	Cefuroxime	306 (52.9%)
	Clindamycin	46 (8.0%)
	Cefuroxime/Metronidazole	24 (4.2%)
	Cefazolin/Metronidazole	15 (2.6%)
III	Cefazolin	21 (5.3%)
	Cefuroxime	195 (49.1%)
	Clindamycin	28 (7.1%)
	Gentamicin	31 (7.8%)
	Cefuroxime/Metronidazole	82 (20.7)
	Cefazolin/Metronidazole	40 (10.1%)

The results of all wound cultures were positive in 552 patients (55.9%). The positivity rates were 48.7% and 70.0% for grades II and III open fractures, respectively (Table 2). Coagulase-negative staphylococci were the most commonly isolated pathogens (37.5%) in grade II open fractures, and *Staphylococcus aureus* was the most commonly isolated pathogen (37.1%) in grade III open fractures. The other commonly isolated pathogens in grade II open fractures were *Staphylococcus aureus* (21.7%), *Pseudomonas aeruginosa* (9.9%), *Enterobacter cloacae* (7.7%), *Acinetobacter baumannii* (7.0%), *Escherichia coli* (5.9%), and group B streptococci (3.7%). The other commonly isolated pathogens in grade III open fractures included coagulase-negative staphylococci (23.7%), *Pseudomonas aeruginosa* (10.1%), *Acinetobacter baumannii* (8.6%), and *Escherichia coli* (6.8%). Six cases of grade III open fractures had polymicrobial wound contamination (2.2%). Anaerobic strains were found in one patient with grade II open fractures and three patients with grade III open fractures. (Table 3)

Table 2. The number of open fractures, microbiological samples, and positive results according to the Gustilo-Anderson classification.

Gustilo-Anderson Classification	Number of Patients	Number of Microbiological Samples	Number of Isolated Pathogens
I	373	32	2
II	578	558	272
III	397	397	290 *

* Polymicrobial wound contamination was found in six patients with III open fractures, which included: *Staphylococcus epidermidis/Pseudomonas aeruginosa, Staphylococcus capotis/Acinetobacter baumannii, Staphylococcus epidermidis/Escherichia coli, Pseudomonas aeruginosa/Enterococcus faecium, Staphylococcus aureus/Acinetobacter baumannii,* and *Staphylococcus aureus/Enterobacter cloaca*.

Table 3. The number of isolated pathogens according to the Gustilo-Anderson classification.

	COST *	Staphylococcus Aureus	Pseudomonas Aeruginosa	Enterobacter Cloacae	Acinetobacter Baumannii	Escherichia coli	Streptococcus B	Enterococcus Faecium	Corynebacterium Jekeium	Anaerobic Strains **	Others ***
I	2	0	0	0	0	0	0	0	0	0	0
II	102	59	27	21	19	16	10	9	7	1	1
III	66	103	28	13	24	19	13	13	6	3	2

* COST: coagulase-negative staphylococci. ** Anaerobic strains: clostridium perfringens. *** Others include *Klebsiella pneumonia* and *Pseudomonas stutzeri*.

Most pathogens, except *Pseudomonas aeruginosa, Enterobacter cloacae*, and *Acinetobacter baumannii*, were sensitive to the prophylactic antibiotics according to the EAST guidelines [5]. We found Gram-negative strains in 83 (30.5%) of grade II open fractures and 84 (30.2%) of grade III open fractures. Among the Gram-negative strains, 21 strains were against gentamicin (12.6%) and 30 against ciprofloxacin (18.0%). We also found 95 problematic Gram-positive strains in grades II and III open fractures that were resistant to first-generation and second-generation cephalosporins and aminopenicillins. Twenty-one of these 45 strains (46.7%) were also not susceptible to gentamicin. (Table 4)

Table 4. Resistance of the isolated pathogens according to the Gustilo-Anderson classification.

Gustilo–Anderson Classification	Isolated Pathogens	n	Resistance	n
I	*Staphylococcus epidermidis*	2	-	-
II	*Staphylococcus epidermidis*	67	Cefazolin	23
			Cefuroxime	28
			Gentamicin	5
			Penicillin	34
			Cotrimoxazole	29
			Amoxicillin Clavulan acid	21
			Tetracycline	27
	Staphylococcus capitis	35	Penicillin	16
			Gentamicin	35
			Cotrimoxazole	35
			Oxacillin	35
			Clindamycin	35
			Fosfomycin	9
	Staphylococcus aureus	59	Penicillin	11
			Cefazolin	16
			Cefuroxime	18
			Levofloxacin	8
			Ciprofloxacin	9
			Gentamicin	3
			Clindamycin	4
			Moxifloxacin	6
			Tetracycline	2
			Amoxicillin clavulan acid	4
	Pseudomonas aeruginosa	27	Cefperazone–sulbactam	11
			Gentamicin	2
			Levofloxacin	6
			Ciprofloxacin	6
			Imipenem	13
			Cefepime	19
			Cefazolin	19
			Cefuroxime	14
	Enterobacter cloacae	21	Imipenem	16
			Aztreonam	18
			Cefperazone–sulbactam	6
			Ceftazidime	19
			Cefepime	18
			Gentamicin	7
			Ceftriaxone	20
			Levofloxacin	9
	Acinetobacter baumannii	19	Ciprofloxacin	14
			Moxifloxacin	15
			Ceftazidime	15
			Imipenem	13
			Cefepime	16
			Ceftriaxone	16
			Cotrimoxazole	11

Table 4. *Cont.*

Gustilo–Anderson Classification	Isolated Pathogens	n	Resistance	n
	Escherichia coli	16	Cefuroxime	12
			Amoxicillin clavulan acid	11
			Imipenem	9
			Ceftazidime	13
			Cefepime	13
			Cefperazone–sulbactam	15
			Ceftriaxone	16
			Gentamicin	5
			Ampicillin	10
	Streptococcus B	10	Tetracycline	5
			Gentamicin	3
	Enterococcus faecium	9	Cefuroxime	9
			Gentamicin	4
			Ciprofloxacin	9
			Moxifloxacin	9
			Cotrimoxazole	1
			Rifampicin	9
			Vancomycin	1
			Tetracycline	3
			Levofloxacin	2
			Ampicillin	1
	Corynebacterium jekeium	7	Ceftazidime	7
			Penicillin	7
			Cefepime	7
			Fosfomycin	6
			Ciprofloxacin	6
			Moxifloxacin	6
			Cotrimoxazole	1
	Clostridium perfringens	1	Penicillin	1
			Aztreonam	1
			Amoxicillin clavulan acid	1
			Tetracycline	1
			Piperacillin	1
			Azithromycin	1
	Klebsiella pneumonia	1	Imipenem	1
			Tigecycline	1
			Cefperazone–sulbactam	1
III			Levofloxacin	1
	Staphylococcus epidermidis	45	Cefazolin	26
			Cefuroxime	26
			Gentamicin	3
			Penicillin	38
			Amoxicillin clavulan acid	16
			Tetracycline	39
			Cotrimoxazole	35
	Staphylococcus capitis	21	Oxacillin	21
			Penicillin	15
			Fosfomycin	7
			Gentamicin	21
			Cotrimoxazole	21
			Clindamycin	21
	Staphylococcus aureus	103	Penicillin	39
			Cefazolin	22
			Cefuroxime	22
			Levofloxacin	16
			Ciprofloxacin	17
			Gentamicin	7

Table 4. *Cont.*

Gustilo–Anderson Classification	Isolated Pathogens	n	Resistance	n
			Clindamycin	6
			Moxifloxacin	16
			Vancomycin	2
			Tetracycline	14
			Amoxicillin clavulan acid	11
	Pseudomonas aeruginosa	28	Cefperazone–sulbactam	13
			Piperacillin–yazobactam	1
			Gentamicin	3
			Levofloxacin	7
			Ciprofloxacin	7
			Imipenem	14
			Cefepime	20
			Cefazolin	20
			Cefuroxime	19
	Enterobacter cloacae	13	Imipenem	3
			Aztreonam	5
			Cefperazone–sulbactam	6
			Ceftazidime	11
			Cefepime	11
			Ceftriaxone	12
			Levofloxacin	5
	Acinetobacter baumannii	24	Ciprofloxacin	3
			Ceftazidime	12
			Cefepime	12
			Ceftriaxone	12
			Cotrimoxazole	4
	Escherichia coli	19	Cefuroxime	13
			Amoxicillin clavulan acid	13
			Levofloxacin	2
			Ceftazidime	13
			Cefepime	13
			Cefperazone–sulbactam	19
			Ceftriaxone	15
			Gentamicin	4
			Ampicillin	11
	Streptococcus B	13	Tetracycline	8
			Gentamicin	4
	Enterococcus faecium	13	Cefuroxime	13
			Ciprofloxacin	13
			Moxifloxacin	13
			Cotrimoxazole	1
			Ampicillin	1
			Rifampicin	13
			Vancomycin	1
			Tetracycline	4
			Levofloxacin	2
	Corynebacterium jekeium	6	Ceftazidime	6
			Cefepime	6
			Fosfomycin	6
			Ciprofloxacin	6
			Moxifloxacin	6
			Cotrimoxazole	1
	Clostridium perfringens	3	Penicillin	3
			Aztreonam	3
			Amoxicillin clavulan acid	3
			Tetracycline	3
			Piperacillin	3
			Azithromycin	3

Table 4. *Cont.*

Gustilo–Anderson Classification	Isolated Pathogens	n	Resistance	n
	Klebsiella pneumonia	1	Imipenem	1
			Tigecycline	1
			Levofloxacin	1
			Cefperazone–sulbactam	1
	Pseudomonas stutzeri	1	Ceftazidime	1
			Cefperazone–sulbactam	1
			Ceftriaxone	1
			Levofloxacin	1

4. Discussion

Infections and complications remain major obstacles to the treatment of open fractures of the lower extremities [5–8]. Our multicenter study was a retrospective study based on six trauma centers in East China, including the Shanghai Jiao Tong University affiliated Sixth People's Hospital (Shanghai, China), the Xiamen University affiliated Fuzhou Second Hospital (Fuzhou, China), the first affiliated hospital of Soochow University (Suzhou, China), the Tongde Hospital of Zhejiang Province (Hangzhou, China), the Second Hospital of Anhui Medical University (Hefei, China), and Shandong Provincial Hospital (Jinan, China).

To our knowledge, this is the first study focusing on the bacterial spectrum and resistance patterns in a cohort of patients with open fractures in East China. The recommended EAST antibiotic prophylaxis guidelines were published in 2000 on the EAST website. Based on a review of 54 articles published from 1975 to 1997, the workgroup offered three level I and two level II recommendations specific to the choice of antibiotic coverage and duration of therapy; the EAST guidelines were updated in 2011 [9,10]. Systemic antibiotic coverage directed at Gram-positive organisms and initiated as soon as possible after an injury is recommended. Additional Gram-negative coverage should be added for grade III open fractures. The EAST guidelines for antibiotic prophylaxis were followed at two of our trauma centers.

According to our results, the bacterial spectrum in the grade II open fractures differed from that of the grade III open fractures; in total, 37.5% of cultures revealed coagulase-negative staphylococci in grade II open fractures and 23.7% in grade III open fractures. The rate of Staphylococcus aureus infection increased from grade II to grade III open fractures. The overall incidences of infections with Gram-positive strains were higher than previously reported from European countries [11–13], which can be explained by the fact that four of our trauma centers did not follow the EAST guidelines. The major problem among these four trauma centers was the delayed administration of prophylactic antibiotics. Lack et al., found lower rates of infection when patients received antibiotics <66 min after injury [11]. No details regarding door-to-antibiotic administration time were available in our study, but they were mostly longer than 4 h according to trauma surgeons in these four centers.

Of significance, the incidence of Gram-negative infections has been increasing in China in the past few years. According to the results of our study, the incidences of Gram-negative bacilli infections in open fractures in grades II and III were around 30.5%. This incidence was relatively high when compared to that reported from Germany, which was as low as 11% [13]. These pathogens isolated from grade II open fractures would not have been adequately covered even if the EAST guidelines were followed, in addition to the other four trauma centers that did not follow the EAST guidelines. Among all the isolated Gram-negative bacteria, nosocomial strains, such as *Pseudomonas aeruginosa*, *Acinetobacter baumannii*, and *Enterococcus faecium*, had surprisingly high incidences (>20%). This may be attributable to several factors, including the limited trauma care workforce, the lack of well-established treatment protocols for severe open fractures, and the failure to strictly follow the guidelines regarding antibiotic prophylaxis.

One patient with grade II open fractures and three patients with grade III open fractures were infected with anaerobic strains, possibly due to heavily soiled wounds. Heavily soiled wounds would be problematic in severe open fractures due to the potentially increasing load of anaerobic bacteria and the common use of cephalosporins with low levels of activity against anaerobic pathogens.

We found 45 problematic Gram-positive strains in grades II and III open fractures that were resistant to first- and second-generation cephalosporins and aminopenicillins. The lowest rates of resistance were identified among strains treated with quinolones, followed by cotrimoxazole. The fluoroquinolones were suspected of having a negative effect on bone healing; no advantage of fluoroquinolones was found compared with a combination regimen of a cephalosporin and an aminoglycoside recommended by the EAST guidelines [10,14,15]. Furthermore, the relatively small proportion prohibits general recommendations.

The positivity rates of the samples obtained from grade III open fractures were 70.0%, which was higher than that of the samples obtained from grade II open fractures. This result can be explained by the fact that high-velocity injuries often result in poor tissue oxygenation and the devitalization of soft tissue and bone. This produces a perfect medium for bacterial multiplication and infection. Accordingly, the greater the volume of involvement of the soft tissue bed in the injury, the easier it is for bacterial multiplication and infection to occur.

Our data highlighted the different characteristics of contamination based on the Gustilo-Anderson classification of open fractures. Wounds from grade III open fractures are more easily contaminated with Staphylococcus aureus compared to those from grade II open fractures. Antibiotic prophylaxis has to be effective against mostly Gram-positive bacteria. Nosocomial infections are mostly due to Gram-negative and drug-resistant strains and usually occur among patients on prolonged treatment with extended exposure times to wounds in trauma centers.

Due to the obstacles in the interhospital exchange of diagnosis and treatment information in China, it has become difficult to collect statistics on the strains of bacteria causing open fractures and their drug resistance. Therefore, it is necessary for the relevant national agencies to intervene and establish a database of information related to open fractures that can be updated in real time with the common strains and their drug resistance. Additionally, guidelines need to be developed and implemented in hospitals at all levels.

The major limitation of this study was the limited number of patients included and the even lower number of patients for whom microbiological samples were initially taken. Most of the trauma centers in our multicenter study lacked a standard protocol for antibiotic prophylaxis and wound sampling. In addition, some of the samples in our study (8%) were taken via swabs, which only represented the microbial colonization of the wound or surrounding skin rather than pathogens causing deep-tissue infections. A lower number of samples may cause difficulties in interpretation, and a higher number would lead to an increased probability of contamination without evidence of the improved sensitivity of the examination.

5. Conclusions

The spectrum of bacteria infecting patients with open fractures is changing in East China. The incidence of nosocomial infection seems to be increasing not only among patients with grade III open fractures but also among those with grade II open fractures. The updated EAST guidelines for antibiotic prophylaxis in open fracture (2011) have been proven to be adequate for a large portion of patients in the USA and most countries in Europe; they have also been proven to be clinically instructive in East China.

Author Contributions: Conceptualization, C.H. and Y.C.; methodology, S.L.; software, S.L.; formal analysis, W.Z.; formal analysis, Y.S.; resources, Y.W. and Y.C.; data curation, H.W. and P.H.; writing—original draft preparation, W.Z.; writing—review and editing, C.H.; visualization, S.L.; supervision, Y.C. and C.H.; project administration, C.H.; funding acquisition, Y.C and C.H. All authors have read and agreed to the published version of the manuscript.

Funding: This research was funded by the National Natural Science Foundation of China, grant number 82203903; the Interdisciplinary Program of Shanghai Jiao Tong University, grant number YG2022QN088; and the Basic Research Project of Shanghai Sixth People's Hospital, grant number YNQN202103.

Institutional Review Board Statement: The study protocol was approved by the Ethics Committee of Shanghai Jiao Tong University Affiliated Sixth People's Hospital, Approval No: 2016-88-(1). Informed consent was obtained from all participants. All study methods were in accordance with the Declaration of Helsinki.

Informed Consent Statement: Informed consent was obtained from all subjects involved in the study.

Data Availability Statement: Data are available upon request due to restrictions on privacy. The data presented in this study are available upon request from the corresponding author.

Conflicts of Interest: The authors declare no conflict of interest.

References

1. Uçkay, I.; Harbarth, S.; Peter, R.; Lew, D.; Hoffmeyer, P.; Pittet, D. Preventing surgical site infections. *Expert Rev. Anti-Infect. Ther.* **2010**, *8*, 657–670. [CrossRef] [PubMed]
2. Abukhder, M.; Dobbs, T.; Shaw, J.; Whelan, R.; Jones, E. A systematic literature review and narrative synthesis on the risk factors for developing affective disorders in open lower-limb fracture patients. *Ann. Med. Surg.* **2022**, *80*, 104190. [CrossRef] [PubMed]
3. Kobata, S.I.; Teixeira, L.E.M.; Fernandes, S.O.A.; Faraco, A.A.G.; Vidigal, P.V.T.; De Araújo, I.D. Prevention of bone infection after open fracture using a chitosan with ciprofloxacin implant in animal model. *Acta Cir. Bras.* **2020**, *35*, e202000803. [CrossRef] [PubMed]
4. Laxminarayan, R.; Duse, A.; Wattal, C.; Zaidi, A.K.M.; Wertheim, H.F.L.; Sumpradit, N.; Vlieghe, E.; Hara, G.L.; Gould, I.M.; Goossens, H.; et al. Antibiotic resistance—The need for global solutions. *Lancet Infect. Dis.* **2013**, *13*, 1057–1098. [CrossRef] [PubMed]
5. Deemer, A.R.; Drake, J.H.; Littlefield, C.P.; Egol, K.A. Surgeon Volume Impacts Outcomes Following Ankle Fracture Repair. *Foot Ankle Orthop.* **2022**, *7*, 24730114221116790. [CrossRef] [PubMed]
6. Williams, J.; Davies, M.; Guduri, V.; Din, A.; Ahluwalia, R. The multi-ligament ankle fracture: Epidemiology, key anatomical findings and fixation strategies in unstable open injuries. *J. Clin. Orthop. Trauma* **2022**, *36*, 102086. [CrossRef] [PubMed]
7. Hake, M.E.; Young, H.; Hak, D.J.; Stahel, P.F.; Hammerberg, E.M.; Mauffrey, C. Local antibiotic therapy strategies in orthopaedic trauma: Practical tips and tricks and review of the literature. *Injury* **2015**, *46*, 1447–1456. [CrossRef] [PubMed]
8. Phaff, M.; Aird, J.; Rollinson, P. Delayed implants sepsis in HIV-positive patients following open fractures treated with orthopaedic implants. *Injury* **2015**, *46*, 590–594. [CrossRef] [PubMed]
9. Luchette, F.A.; Borzotta, A.P.; Croce, M.A.; O'Neill, P.A.; Whittmann, D.H.; Mullins, C.D.; Palumbo, F.; Pasquale, M.D. Practice Management Guidelines for Prophylactic Antibiotic Use in Penetrating Abdominal Trauma: The EAST Practice Management Guidelines Work Group. *J. Trauma Inj. Infect. Crit. Care* **2000**, *48*, 508–518. [CrossRef] [PubMed]
10. Hoff, W.S.; Bonadies, J.A.; Cachecho, R.; Dorlac, W.C. East Practice Management Guidelines Work Group: Update to Practice Management Guidelines for Prophylactic Antibiotic Use in Open Fractures. *J. Trauma Inj. Infect. Crit. Care* **2011**, *70*, 751–754. [CrossRef] [PubMed]
11. Lack, W.D.; Karunakar, M.A.; Angerame, M.R.; Seymour, R.B.; Sims, S.; Kellam, J.F.; Bosse, M.J. Type III open tibia fractures: Immediate antibiotic prophylaxis minimizes infection. *J. Orthop. Trauma* **2015**, *29*, 1–6. [CrossRef] [PubMed]
12. Johnson, H.C.; Bailey, A.M.; Baum, R.A.; Justice, S.B.; Weant, K.A. Compliance and Related Outcomes of Prophylactic Antibiotics in Traumatic Open Fractures. *Hosp. Pharm.* **2020**, *55*, 193–198. [CrossRef] [PubMed]
13. Otchwemah, R.; Grams, V.; Tjardes, T.; Shafizadeh, S.; Bäthis, H.; Maegele, M.; Messler, S.; Bouillon, B.; Probst, C. Bacterial contamination of open fractures—Pathogens, antibiotic resistances and therapeutic regimes in four hospitals of the trauma network Cologne, Germany. *Injury* **2015**, *46* (Suppl. 4), S104–S108. [CrossRef] [PubMed]
14. James, K.C.; Alexander, L.A.; Sharon, R.L. Timing of antibiotic administration, wound debridement, and the stages of reconstructive surgery for open long bone fractures of the upper and lower limbs. *Cochrane Database Syst. Rev.* **2022**, *4*, CD013555. [CrossRef]
15. Willem-Jan, M.; Austin, T.F.; TFintan, M. Evidence-Based Recommendations for Local Antimicrobial Strategies and Dead Space Management in Fracture-Related Infection. *J. Orthop. Trauma* **2020**, *34*, 18–29. [CrossRef]

Disclaimer/Publisher's Note: The statements, opinions and data contained in all publications are solely those of the individual author(s) and contributor(s) and not of MDPI and/or the editor(s). MDPI and/or the editor(s) disclaim responsibility for any injury to people or property resulting from any ideas, methods, instructions or products referred to in the content.

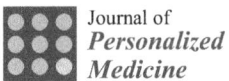

Article

Intra-Articular Injection of Autologous Micro-Fragmented Adipose Tissue for the Treatment of Knee Osteoarthritis: A Prospective Interventional Study

Yang Yu [1,2,†], Qunshan Lu [1,†], Songlin Li [1,3], Mingxing Liu [4], Houyi Sun [1], Lei Li [1,2], Kaifei Han [1,2] and Peilai Liu [1,*]

1. Department of Orthopaedics, Qilu Hospital of Shandong University, Jinan 250102, China
2. Cheeloo College of Medicine, Shandong University, Jinan 250012, China
3. Chinese Academy of Medical Sciences and Peking Union Medical College, Beijing 100730, China
4. Boshan District Hospital of Traditional Chinese Medicine, Zibo 255200, China
* Correspondence: 199362000205@mail.sdu.edu.cn
† These authors contributed equally to this work.

Abstract: Background: To investigate the efficacy and safety of autologous micro-fragmented adipose tissue (MF-AT) for improving joint function and cartilage repair in patients with knee osteoarthritis. Methods: From March 2019 to December 2020, 20 subjects (40 knees) between 50 and 65 years old suffering from knee osteoarthritis were enrolled in the study and administered a single injection of autologous MF-A. The data of all patients were prospectively collected. The Western Ontario and McMaster Universities Osteoarthritis Index (WOMAC), knee society score (KSS), hospital for special surgery (HSS) score, visual analogue score (VAS) pain score, changes in cartilage Recht grade on magnetic resonance imaging (MRI) and adverse events were analyzed before and 3, 6, 9, 12 and 18 months after injection. Results: The WOMAC, VAS, KSS and HSS scores at 3, 6, 9, 12 and 18 months after injection were improved compared with those before injection ($p < 0.05$). There was no significant difference in WOMAC scores between 9 and 12 months after injection ($p > 0.05$), but the WOMAC score 18 months after injection was worse than that at the last follow-up ($p < 0.05$). The VAS, KSS and HSS scores 9, 12 and 18 months after injection were worse than those at the last follow-up ($p < 0.05$). The Recht score improvement rate was 25%. No adverse events occurred during the follow-up. Conclusions: Autologous MF-AT improves knee function and relieves pain with no adverse events. However, the improved knee function was not sustained, with the best results occurring 9–12 months after injection and the cartilage regeneration remaining to be investigated.

Keywords: knee osteoarthritis; micro-fragmented adipose tissue; cartilage repair; mesenchymal stem cells

1. Introduction

Osteoarthritis (OA) is a kind of joint degenerative disease caused by many factors and leads to irreversible cartilage damage, subchondral osteosclerosis and synovitis [1]. It is caused by degeneration of articular cartilage and subchondral bone. According to a previous survey, approximately 9.6% of men and 18% of women over the age of 60 years suffer from symptomatic OA worldwide [2]. Currently, many treatment modalities for knee OA, such as lifestyle modification and pharmaceuticals, are advocated [3]. However, advanced knee OA eventually requires joint surgery as the disease progresses [2,4,5]. It is still unknown how to reverse the progression of osteoarthritis of the knee.

Micro-fragmented adipose tissue (MF-AT) is composed of three-dimensional biological scaffolds and colonies of cells in which the three-dimensional biological scaffolds are composed of collagen and connective tissue and microvascular networks, and the clustered cells consist of pericytes, adipocytes and MSCs, among others [6]. Mesenchymal stem cells (MSCs) are pluripotent stem cells that have the potential to self-renew and to multidifferentiate in a variety of tissues in the body [7]. With characteristics of easy expansion,

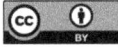

self-renewal, multidiversification and low immunogenicity, they are usually derived from adipose tissue, umbilical cord blood or bone marrow [8–11]. Studies have shown that intra-articular injections of MSCs can treat cartilage in the knee [11]. The adipose mesenchymal stem cells (AD-MSCs) contained in autologous MF-AT are one of the many MSCs that have the ability to differentiate into articular chondrocytes. In addition, more than 100 kinds of cytokines have been detected to endow MF-AT with strong antibacterial, anti-inflammatory and antiapoptotic properties that promote vascular regeneration and tissue repair [12]. Although previous studies have confirmed the effectiveness of intra-articular injection of autologous MF-AT for knee OA, the effective time and administration interval of MF-AT remain to be explored.

Therefore, we conducted a prospective interventional study to evaluate the change in clinical effect over time of intra-articular injection of autologous MF-AT and their effect on cartilage repair in patients with knee OA. The purpose of this study is as follows: 1. the effect and duration of autologous MF-AT on functional recovery of the knee joint; 2. the effect on the repair of cartilage; and 3. its safety.

2. Materials and Methods

2.1. Study Design

The study is a single-center, interventional, prospective, interventional study (NCT 03956719). The study protocol was approved by the Ethics Committee of Qilu Hospital of Shandong University (KYLL-2018-023), and all participants provided written informed consent.

2.2. Patient Selection

From March 2019 to December 2020, patients were recruited from an outpatient clinic because of symptomatic knee osteoarthritis, and the first eligible outpatient per month was included. The inclusion criteria of the study were as follows: (1) patients aged between 50 and 65 years, and an American Society of Anesthesiologists (ASA) score from grade one to grade three; (2) patients with bilateral knee OA; and (3) patients with a Recht grade 1–3 on MRI. The exclusion criteria were as follows: (1) patients with acute joint injury, knee joint tuberculosis, tumor or rheumatic diseases; (2) pregnant or lactating women; (3) patients with an allergic constitution; (4) patients who underwent other knee surgery performed within 6 months; (5) those who had incomplete data affecting the efficacy or safety judgment; or (6) subjects who could not understand and voluntarily sign the written informed consent or comply with the research protocol and visitation process.

2.3. Surgical Procedure

The procedure was performed at the same place by the same specialized physician who was not involved in any of the evaluations of the participants. Autologous MF-AT was prepared using a Lipogems® device (Lipogems International SpA, Milan, Italy). A Lipogems® device is a device specifically used for liposuction and adipose tissue treatment. It can obtain pure autologous MF-AT through physical manipulation [13]. In this way, the product containing pericytes is retained within an intact stromal vascular niche and interacts with the recipient tissue after transplantation, thereby becoming activated as MSCs [14,15]. All patients were operated on in a randomized sequence.

After local anesthesia and sterilization were successfully induced, the swelling solution (composed of 500 mL normal saline, 50 mL lidocaine (2%) and 1 mL adrenaline (1:1000)) was injected into the extraction site. The gas in the device was emptied and the clamps at both ends of the device were closed. Then, liposuction was carried out at the premarked area with a vacuum syringe. The amount of adipose tissue mixture was generally 80–100 mL (Figure 1). The wound was covered with a dressing and the abdominal band was bandaged and fixed for 3 days. The next step is to manipulate the adipose tissue. Adipose tissue was injected into the device from the inlet, the outlet clamp was opened and 1/3 of the volume of the device was injected. The inlet clamp was opened, and flushing began. The clamps were closed at both ends, and vibration was performed for 30 s. The above operation was then repeated 4 times. During the washing process, lidocaine, blood, grease, etc., were removed and the autologous MF-AT was obtained. After washing, the clamp was closed at both ends, the device was turned upside down, a 10-mL syringe was connected to both ends of the device and the clamp was opened at the inlet. The syringe was pushed to obtain the autologous MF-AT. The autologous MF-AT was then injected into the knee joint. The patient should flex and extend the knee joint to ensure that the MF-AT are evenly distributed within the joint.

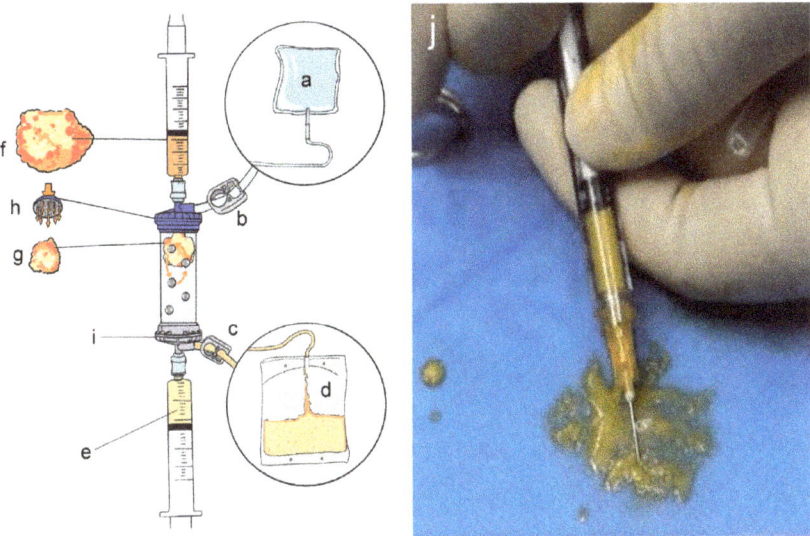

Figure 1. Lipogems® device and autologous micro-fragmented adipose tissue. (**a**): Physiological saline bag (3–5 L); (**b**): inlet clamp; (**c**): outlet clamp; (**d**): waste bag: collection of oils and blood residues; (**e**): final products; (**f**): pristine adipose tissue; (**g**): adipose tissue after shaking and emulsification; (**h**): primitive adipose tissue entry; (**i**): final product collection port; (**j**): autologous micro-fragmented adipose tissue.

The autologous MF-AT were extracted intraoperatively and injected rapidly into the patient, so we did not quantitatively count the AD-MSCs injected into the patient but controlled for the volume of the fragment. After removing other impurities through the Lipogems® device, the injection volume of all patients in this study was 6–8 mL per knee joint. The entire procedure lasted approximately 30 min. Because the damage caused by this surgery was very small and it was strictly performed aseptically, we did not use prophylactic antibiotics to prevent infection. One day after the operation, if there was no discomfort, the patient was discharged from the hospital.

2.4. Outcome Measures

Basic information such as patient age, sex, height, weight, body mass index (BMI), disease duration and preoperative comorbidities (e.g., diabetes, hypertension) were recorded. The Western Ontario and McMaster Universities (WOMAC) score, hospital for special surgery (HSS) score, knee society score (KSS) and visual analogue scale (VAS) pain score were recorded preoperatively 1 month, 3 months, 6 months, 9 months, 12 months and 18 months after the operation. All data were recorded by the same researcher who did not participate in the operation. See Figure 2 for details.

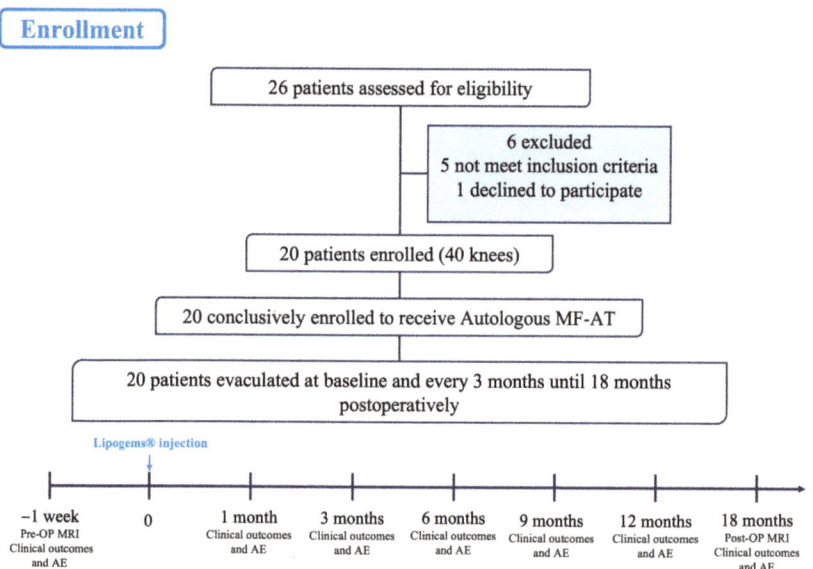

Figure 2. Flow chart of the clinical trial. MF-AT: micro-fragmented adipose tissue; AE: adverse events.

The degree of cartilage injury under magnetic resonance imaging evaluation (MRI) was described by Recht grading [16]. MRI was performed using a 3.0-T scanner with an 8-channel knee coil. The maximum gradient strength was 80 mT/m, while the maximum slew rate was 100 mT/m/ms. The thickness and spacing of the scanning layer were 3.0 mm and 0.6 mm, respectively. The images were digitally transmitted to the image archiving and communication system. Radiological measurements were made using the electronic calipers and goniometers provided with the software. The evaluations were performed by a senior radiologist who was blinded to the patient's information.

Patients were considered to have postejection adverse events when they experienced hypersensitivity, fever, nausea and vomiting, cardiovascular events, severe pain, bleeding, marked swelling, surgical site infection and infection of the knee joint.

2.5. Statistical Analysis

The sample size was performed with PASS 2011 (NCSS, LLC, Kaysville, UT, USA) and calculated using WOMAC as the primary outcome. A difference of 10 points was assumed during the follow-up period ($\alpha = 0.05$; $\beta = 0.80$). Considering an intra-group standard deviation of 15 points, 16 subjects were needed to obtain the required statistical power. Considering a 15% dropout rate, the minimum sample size was 19 cases. Statistical analysis was performed with SPSS version 26 (IBM, New York, NY, USA) and GraphPad Prism version 8 (GraphPad Software, San Diego, CA, USA). Continuous variables are subject to normal distribution based on the Shapiro–Wilk test. Continuous variables were reported as means and standard errors. Paired sample t-tests were used to test if there was a statistically significant difference between the two groups. Categorical variables were recorded as incidence and rate. All statistical tests were performed with bilateral tests, and p values less than or equal to 0.05 were considered statistically significant.

3. Results

3.1. Demographic Characteristics

A total of 20 patients with knee OA (40 knees) were included in this experiment. The 20 patients comprised 12 females and 8 males aged 54.63 ± 3.90 years (49–60 years), with a mean BMI of approximately 25.5 ± 2.86 kg/m^2 (21.3–28.76 kg/m$_2$). All of them had a history of knee OA for more than 2 years (6.9 ± 3.2 years) and received conservative treatment without surgery during this period, and the degree of lower limb coronal alignment was 12.58 ± 3.59° (5.5–18.0°). Seven patients had hypertension and four had type II diabetes mellitus. The remaining patients had no concomitant chronic diseases. See Table 1 for details.

Table 1. Demographic characteristics of the patients.

	Values
Patients (n)	20
Knees (n)	40
Age (years)	55 ± 3.9
Sex (n, %)	
Male	8 (40%)
Female	12 (60%)
Height (cm)	165 ± 0.05
Weight (kg)	69.3 ± 8.48
Body mass index (kg/m^2)	25.5 ± 2.86
Symptom duration (years)	6.9 ± 3.2
Lower limb alignment (varus angle°)	12.58 ± 3.59
Baseline knee function	
WOMAC score	24.87 ± 15.44
VAS	4.20 ± 1.42
KSS	77.73 ± 11.71
HSS score	79.73 ± 8.91
Comorbidities	AHT in 7 patients (35%) DM in 4 patients (20%)

Abbreviations: WOMAC: the Western Ontario and McMaster Universities Osteoarthritis Index; VAS: visual analogue score; KSS: knee society score; HSS: hospital for special surgery; AHT: arterial hypertension; DM: diabetes mellitus.

3.2. Knee Function Outcomes

3.2.1. WOMAC Score

At the last follow-up, the WOMAC scores of 20 patients after injection were improved ($p < 0.05$) from 24.87 ± 1.44 before injection to 17.13 ± 12.33 18 months after injection. The WOMAC score of 20 patients decreased continuously from before injection to 3 months, 6 months and 9 months after injection ($p < 0.05$). The scores at 9 months and 12 months after injection were compared ($p > 0.05$) (Table 2 (A and B)), and the results indicated that there was no significant difference between 9 months and 12 months after injection. From 12 months to 18 months after injection, the score began to increase (from 7.93 ± 6.44 to 17.13 ± 12.33, as shown in Figure 3 and Table 2 (A and B)), and there was a significant difference between the two scores ($p < 0.05$). These data indicate that the 20 patients had the best knee function at 9–12 months after the application of MF-AT. See Table 2 and Figure 3 for details.

Table 2. Changes in knee joint function outcomes during follow-up.

A. WOMAC Score Comparison between Adjacent Follow-Up Periods

WOMAC score	Baseline	1 month	3 months	6 months	9 months	12 months	18 months
Mean	24.87	19.33	13.87	10.00	7.40	7.93	17.13
SD	15.44	11.68	8.70	7.04	5.63	6.44	12.33
T		3.517	4.323	6.526	4.516	−0.725	−4.545
p value		0.003	0.001	0.001	0.001	0.481	0.001

B. WOMAC Score Comparison between Specific Time Periods

WOMAC score	Mean	SD	T	p value
Baseline	24.87	15.44	6.380	0.001
9 months	7.40	5.63		
Baseline	24.87	15.44	5.528	0.001
18 months	17.13	12.33		
9 months	7.40	5.63	−4.935	0.001
18 months	17.13	12.33		

C. VAS Comparison between Adjacent Follow-Up Periods

VAS	Baseline	1 month	3 months	6 months	9 months	12 months	18 months
Mean	4.2	3.07	1.8	1.27	0.4	0.87	1.73
SD	1.42	1.33	1.08	0.8	0.63	0.64	0.88
T		5.906	6.141	2.779	5.245	−2.432	−4.516
p value		0.001	0.001	0.015	0.001	0.029	0.001

D. VAS Comparison between Specific Time Periods

VAS	Mean	SD	T	p value
Baseline	4.2	1.42	12.192	0.001
9 months	0.4	0.63		
Baseline	4.2	1.42	9.012	0.001
18 months	1.73	0.88		
9 months	0.4	0.63	−8.367	0.001
18 months	1.73	0.88		

E. KSS Comparison between Adjacent Follow-Up Periods

KSS	Baseline	1 month	3 months	6 months	9 months	12 months	18 months
Mean	77.73	83.27	89.4	93.53	95.93	95.2	90.6
SD	11.71	12.12	7.9	6.03	4.54	4.23	6.49
T		−8.98	−3.992	−5.141	−3.032	1.661	6.2
p value		0.001	0.001	0.001	0.009	0.119	0.001

F. KSS Comparison between Specific Time Periods

KSS	Mean	SD	T	p value
Baseline	77.73	11.71	−8.684	0.001
9 months	95.93	4.54		
Baseline	77.73	11.71	−6.940	0.001
18 months	90.6	6.49		
9 months	95.93	4.54	6.904	0.001
18 months	90.6	6.49		

G. HSS Score Comparison between Adjacent Follow-Up Periods

HSS score	Baseline	1 month	3 months	6 months	9 months	12 months	18 months
Mean	79.73	86.53	91.33	93.73	95.93	94	89.07
SD	8.91	8.02	6.22	5.52	4.27	5.26	6.98
T		−6.961	−6.339	−4.505	−4.785	2.377	6.396
p value		0.001	0.001	0.001	0.001	0.032	0.001

Table 2. *Cont.*

H. HSS Score Comparison between Specific Time Periods				
HSS score	Mean	SD	T	*p* value
Baseline	79.73	8.91	−9.350	0.001
9 months	95.93	4.27		
Baseline	79.73	8.91	−5.709	0.001
18 months	89.07	6.98		
9 months	95.93	4.27	6.198	0.001
18 months	89.07	6.98		

Abbreviations: WOMAC: the Western Ontario and McMaster Universities; VAS: visual analogue scale; KSS: knee society score; HSS: hospital for special surgery score; SD: standard errors.

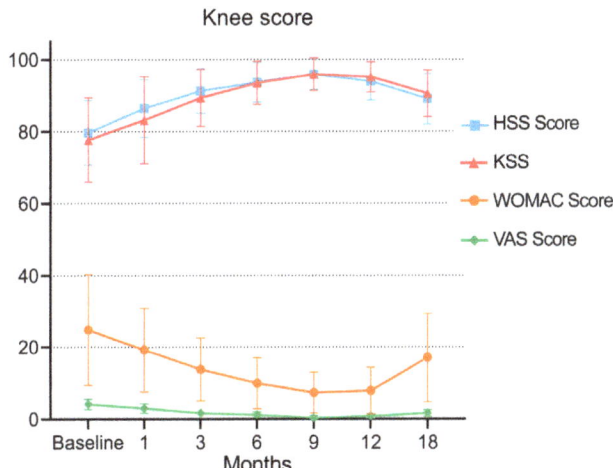

Figure 3. Changes in the WOMAC score, VAS, HSS score and KSS during follow-up.

3.2.2. KSS and HSS Score

After 18 months of follow-up, the KSS of the patients increased from 77.73 ± 11.71 to 90.6 ± 6.49, and the HSS score increased from 79.73 ± 8.91 to 89.07 ± 6.98. There were significant differences between the scores before injection and 18 months after injection ($p < 0.05$, as shown in Table 2 (E–H) and Figure 3). The KSS of the 20 patients increased continuously from before injection to 3 months, 6 months and 9 months after injection (from 77.73 ± 11.71 to 95.93 ± 4.54), as did the HSS score (from 79.73 ± 8.91 to 95.93 ± 4.27). From 9 months to 12 and 18 months after injection, the scores of the two groups gradually decreased (KSS from 95.93 ± 4.54 to 90.6 ± 6.49, HSS score from 95.93 ± 4.27 to 89.07 ± 6.98, as shown in Table 2 (E and G) and Figure 3), and the scores at each follow-up were worse than those at the last follow-up ($p < 0.05$). See Table 2 and Figure 3 for details.

3.2.3. VAS Pain Score

From before injection to 3 months, 6 months and 9 months after injection, the VAS pain score of the patients decreased continuously (from 4.2 ± 1.42 to 0.4 ± 0.63), and there was a significant difference from the score before injection ($p < 0.05$, as shown in Table 2 (C and D) and Figure 3). The VAS pain score gradually increased from 9 months to 12 and 18 months after injection (from 0.4 ± 0.63 to 1.73 ± 0.88, $p < 0.05$). However, 18 months after injection compared with before injection, the score was improved, and there was a significant difference ($p < 0.05$), indicating that 18 months after injection, the patient's pain symptoms were relieved and that the pain symptoms were the mildest and the effect was the best in the ninth month after the application of MF-AT. See Table 2 and Figure 3 for details.

3.3. Radiological Outcomes

Twenty-eight of forty knees were Recht grade II, and twelve were Recht grade III before injection. Eighteen months after injection, eight were Recht grade I, twenty-two were Recht grade II, and ten were Recht grade III. The Recht score improvement rate was 25%. In Supplementary Figure S1, the MRI findings of two patients before and after receiving an intra-articular injection of MF-AT are enumerated. In the coronal and sagittal planes, we could see that the knee oedema was slightly reduced compared with that before the application of MF-AT, but cartilage regeneration was not significant.

3.4. Safety

There were no hypersensitivity, fever, nausea and vomiting, cardiovascular events, severe pain, bleeding, marked swelling, surgical site infection and infection of the knee joint during follow-up. All patients were discharged on the first day after injection.

After the injection of autologous micro-fragmented adipose tissue, knee function gradually improved with the platform period of 9–12 months, and the effect began to decline after 12 months. Score. HSS: hospital for special surgery score; KSS: knee society score; WOMAC: the Western Ontario and McMaster Universities; VAS: visual analogue scale.

4. Discussion

The most important finding of this study is that a single intra-articular injection of MF-AT in patients with knee OA resulted in satisfactory clinical results and functional improvement with no adverse events at the 18-month follow-up, with patients showing the best improvement in knee function by 9 months post-injection.

Knee OA is a chronic progressive degenerative disease that can lead to knee pain and dysfunction and seriously affect daily life, especially in elderly individuals. Pain and loss of function are the main clinical features leading to treatment, including nonpharmacological, pharmacological, and surgical methods [17]. The development and progression of OA is a multifactorial disease, and patients vary greatly in age, BMI and daily activities [18–20]. To date, no treatment can reverse knee degeneration or promote articular cartilage regeneration. However, in the body, MSCs are found mainly in tissues such as the periosteum, synovium, adipose tissue and bone marrow and are suitable cells for repairing damaged tissues; under certain conditions, they can efficiently differentiate into muscle, fat and cartilage and other tissues [11]. Some studies have shown that after intra-articular injection, MSCs attach to cartilage defects, increase in number and participate in the regeneration of articular cartilage [8,21]. Adipose tissue is an easily accessible source of MSCs, and its micro fractionation state MF-AT allows for rapid harvesting of relevant volumes of minimally manipulated tissue consisting of clusters containing MSCs [22]. Furthermore, compared to raw adipose tissue, MF-AT contains fewer leukocytes and supra-adventitial-adipose stromal cells, as well as abundant endothelial progenitor cells, which have been described to maintain proliferation and differentiation in interaction with tissue-resident cells [23].

MSCs are depleted, and their ability to proliferate and differentiate is reduced in the microenvironment of osteoarthritis [24]. Therefore, providing large quantities of healthy and functional MSCs helps promote repair or inhibits the progression of cartilage loss [25]. Adipose tissue is much less expensive and invasive to obtain than bone marrow and is more abundant. In addition, the proliferation rate of MSCs from adipose tissue is higher than that derived from of bone marrow [26]. Lipogems® is a simple system designed to collect, process and transfer refined adipose tissue, with great regenerative potential and optimal processing capacity [13]. The adipose tissue is mechanically shredded and washed until there is no free proinflammatory oil or blood residue, and the resulting product is composed of small intact adipose tissue clusters (250–650 microns) containing pericytes retained in intact interstitial vascular niches [13,27]. The end product MF-AT is injected into the joint cavity and activated as MSCs and begins its regeneration process. Therefore, this product is more widely used clinically. However, clinicians and patients remain concerned about the safety of the product. Lipogems® technology obtains autologous MF-AT after special treatment with autologous fat, which can restore the microenvironment of cell growth to the maximum extent. In theory, these microparticles have been considered safe since they do not lead to the formation of antibodies [28]. There may be a decreased risk of tumorigenesis, disease transmission and host immune rejection compared with the use of allogeneic adipose-derived MSCs [29]. However, in previous studies using allogeneic MSCs for intra-articular injection, few adverse events were reported, and the improvement of clinical symptoms was not greatly different from studies using autologous MSCs [30,31]. Intra-articular injectable allogeneic MSCs still need to undergo further clinical study, including for clinical efficacy and safety. Davatchi et al. conducted a study in 2016 on three patients who were injected with autogenous bone marrow MSCs and followed up for 5 years [32]. The indicators of these three patients significantly improved and then gradually deteriorated six months after injection. However, the knee function was still better than that before injection, and no adverse events occurred in the fifth year. Our results show similar functional changes and we conclude that autologous MF-AT is safe for short-term injection. The follow-up period of this study was 18 months, and no serious adverse events occurred during this time.

After the injection of autologous MF-AT, the expected effect appeared at 3–6 months, the platform period was 9–12 months, and the effect began to decline after 12 months. The patients showed the best improvement in knee function by 9 months post-injection in this study. These data all show that after a single injection of MF-AT, the effect can be maintained for approximately 9 months, with some improvement in patients' pain symptoms and knee function. Therefore, intra-articular injection of autologous MF-AT may be a viable option for the treatment of degenerative osteoarthritis. In addition, there are case reports showing that patients with OA and unresponsive pain in the knee joint associated with meniscal injury treated with intra-articular injections of AD-MSCs have improved joint function [33]. Recently, intra-articular injection of AD-MSCs in one patient with posttraumatic cartilage injury improved knee function [34]. Twelve weeks after injection of AD-MSCs, the Oxford knee score improved from 36 (baseline) to 46, and MRI studies 12 months after injection demonstrated an improved cartilage damage signal. Thirty months after receiving an injection, the patient was able to ski naturally. In the present study, we injected one autologous MF-AT, a blend, within the articular cavity, which was comparable to other studies that independently used MSCs [9,30,35,36] and added a rich cell population, intact three-dimensional bioscaffolds and multiple cell growth factors [8,29,34]. These adjuvants may better sustain the repair of MSCs, relieve pain and improve joint function in patients.

By following up with patients and performing MRI examinations, we were able to intuitively observe the effects of autologous MF-AT on knee cartilage before and after injection at different stages. In several previous studies [10,30,37], similar cartilage changes after intra-articular injection of MSCs in patients with knee OA were reported. These studies measured cartilage by T2 relaxation time and cartilage index. Lee et al. conducted a prospective, double-blind, randomized, controlled phase IIb clinical trial in 2019 in which 12 patients (experimental group) were given AD-MSCs and compared with 12 patients (control group) who received normal saline [11]. The observation time was 6 months, and no obvious changes in cartilage were found in the experimental group at the 6-month follow-up after injection; however, the cartilage defects were significantly increased in the control group. Since the results for the measurement of cartilage volume on MRI are inconclusive internationally, in this study, we judged cartilage changes only by observing the MRI images of the patients, and we did not quantify the cartilage changes. Currently, the T2 mapping technique is considered to have great potential for use in the clinic [38]. The T2 mapping technique can assess cartilage structural integrity, tissue structure and water content by measuring T2 values, which is beneficial for the sensitive measurement of histological changes in cartilage. However, this technique has high sensitivity and low specificity, and the measurement of T2 values is performed manually by clinicians, making it susceptible to subjective effects and unfavorable for early diagnosis. Therefore, T2 mapping sequences have not been widely used in the clinical diagnosis of articular cartilage imaging [39]. In the MRI images before and after the injection, we could observe a partial improvement in the Recht grading of the knee cartilage, but there was no significant evidence of cartilage regeneration. Over time, the effect of autologous MF-AT on cartilage still needs further study.

Our study still had some limitations. First, the sample size of the experiment was small, with only 20 patients (40 knees) participating in the present experiment, and specific individuals had a large effect on the experiment. Second, conclusions regarding efficacy are weak due to the lack of a control group and an inability to compare our patients with patients who did not undergo MF-AT. Third, since MF-AT is a mixed compound, with so many active components, would the activity and effect vary among different people, especially given the differences in age, BMI and daily activity, among other variables. Moreover, autologous MF-AT was extracted intraoperatively and rapidly injected into the patients, so we did not quantify the AD-MSCs injected into the patients. In addition, observation of cartilage regeneration by conventional MRI alone may be inadequate, and methods are needed that can quantitatively assess the volume of cartilage regeneration. Despite these shortcomings, given the limited data on this particular treatment method, we believe this study is a valuable addition to the literature.

5. Conclusions

It has been found that intra-articular injection of autologous MF-AT provided satisfactory functional improvement and pain relief in patients with knee OA and caused no adverse events at the 18-month follow-up. However, the improvement in knee function did not persist, with optimal results occurring 9–12 months after injection, and cartilage regeneration remaining to be discussed. Future prospective multicenter studies with large samples are needed to evaluate the long-term effects of autologous MF-AT in patients with knee OA.

Supplementary Materials: The following supporting information can be downloaded at: https://www.mdpi.com/article/10.3390/jpm13030504/s1, Figure S1: changes in MRI before and after injection of autologous micro-fragmented adipose tissue.

Author Contributions: Conceptualization, P.L.; data curation, Y.Y., S.L. and Q.L.; formal analysis, Y.Y. and M.L.; investigation, Y.Y., H.S., L.L. and K.H.; methodology, S.L.; writing—original draft, Y.Y. and S.L.; writing—review and editing, P.L. and Q.L. All authors have read and agreed to the published version of the manuscript.

Funding: This work was funded by the Rongxiang Regenerative Medicine Foundation of Shandong University (2019SDRX-17), the National Nature Science Foundation of China (NSFC, 82071470) and the Natural Science Foundation of Shandong Province (ZR2020MH278).

Institutional Review Board Statement: This study was approved by the Ethics Committee of Qilu Hospital of Shandong University (KYLL-2018-023).

Informed Consent Statement: Informed consent was obtained from all subjects involved in the study.

Data Availability Statement: The data associated with the paper are not publicly available but are available from the corresponding author upon reasonable request.

Conflicts of Interest: The authors declare no conflict of interest.

References

1. Findlay, D.M. If good things come from above, do bad things come from below? *Arthritis Res. Ther.* **2010**, *12*, 119. [CrossRef]
2. Murray, C.J.L.; Lopez, A.D. *The Global Burden of Disease: A Comprehensive Assessment of Mortality and Disability from Diseases, Injuries, and Risk Factors in 1990 and Projected to 2020*; Harvard School of Public Health on behalf of the World Health Organization and the World Bank: Cambridge, MA, USA, 1996; p. 990.
3. Zhang, Y.; Bi, Q.; Luo, J.; Tong, Y.; Yu, T.; Zhang, Q. The Effect of Autologous Adipose-Derived Stromal Vascular Fractions on Cartilage Regeneration Was Quantitatively Evaluated Based on the 3D-FS-SPGR Sequence: A Clinical Trial Study. *BioMed Res. Int.* **2022**, *2022*, 2777568. [CrossRef] [PubMed]

4. Zhang, W.; Moskowitz, R.W.; Nuki, G.; Abramson, S.; Altman, R.D.; Arden, N.; Bierma-Zeinstra, S.; Brandt, K.D.; Croft, P.; Doherty, M.; et al. OARSI recommendations for the management of hip and knee osteoarthritis, part I: Critical appraisal of existing treatment guidelines and systematic review of current research evidence. *Osteoarthr. Cartil.* **2007**, *15*, 981–1000. [CrossRef] [PubMed]
5. Buttgereit, F.; Burmester, G.R.; Bijlsma, J.W. Non-surgical management of knee osteoarthritis: Where are we now and where do we need to go? *RMD Open* **2015**, *1*, e000027. [CrossRef] [PubMed]
6. Natali, S.; Screpis, D.; Farinelli, L.; Iacono, V.; Vacca, V.; Gigante, A.; Zorzi, C. The use of intra-articular injection of autologous micro-fragmented adipose tissue as pain treatment for ankle osteoarthritis: A prospective not randomized clinical study. *Int. Orthop.* **2021**, *45*, 2239–2244. [CrossRef]
7. Pastides, P.; Chimutengwende-Gordon, M.; Maffulli, N.; Khan, W. Stem cell therapy for human cartilage defects: A systematic review. *Osteoarthr. Cartil.* **2013**, *21*, 646–654. [CrossRef]
8. Lee, K.B.; Hui, J.H.; Song, I.C.; Ardany, L.; Lee, E.H. Injectable mesenchymal stem cell therapy for large cartilage defects–a porcine model. *Stem Cells* **2007**, *25*, 2964–2971. [CrossRef]
9. Lu, L.; Dai, C.; Zhang, Z.; Du, H.; Li, S.; Ye, P.; Fu, Q.; Zhang, L.; Wu, X.; Dong, Y.; et al. Treatment of knee osteoarthritis with intra-articular injection of autologous adipose-derived mesenchymal progenitor cells: A prospective, randomized, double-blind, active-controlled, phase IIb clinical trial. *Stem Cell Res. Ther.* **2019**, *10*, 143. [CrossRef]
10. Jo, C.H.; Chai, J.W.; Jeong, E.C.; Oh, S.; Shin, J.S.; Shim, H.; Yoon, K.S. Intra-articular Injection of Mesenchymal Stem Cells for the Treatment of Osteoarthritis of the Knee: A 2-Year Follow-up Study. *Am. J. Sports Med.* **2017**, *45*, 2774–2783. [CrossRef]
11. Lee, W.S.; Kim, H.J.; Kim, K.I.; Kim, G.B.; Jin, W. Intra-Articular Injection of Autologous Adipose Tissue-Derived Mesenchymal Stem Cells for the Treatment of Knee Osteoarthritis: A Phase IIb, Randomized, Placebo-Controlled Clinical Trial. *Stem Cells Transl. Med.* **2019**, *8*, 504–511. [CrossRef]
12. Malanga, G.A.; Chirichella, P.S.; Hogaboom, N.S.; Capella, T. Clinical evaluation of micro-fragmented adipose tissue as a treatment option for patients with meniscus tears with osteoarthritis: A prospective pilot study. *Int. Orthop.* **2021**, *45*, 473–480. [CrossRef]
13. Tremolada, C.; Colombo, V.; Ventura, C. Adipose Tissue and Mesenchymal Stem Cells: State of the Art and Lipogems® Technology Development. *Curr. Stem Cell Rep.* **2016**, *2*, 304–312. [CrossRef]
14. Randelli, P.; Menon, A.; Ragone, V.; Creo, P.; Bergante, S.; Randelli, F.; De Girolamo, L.; Alfieri Montrasio, U.; Banfi, G.; Cabitza, P.; et al. Lipogems Product Treatment Increases the Proliferation Rate of Human Tendon Stem Cells without Affecting Their Stemness and Differentiation Capability. *Stem Cells Int.* **2016**, *2016*, 4373410. [CrossRef]
15. Mautner, K.; Bowers, R.; Easley, K.; Fausel, Z.; Robinson, R. Functional Outcomes Following Microfragmented Adipose Tissue Versus Bone Marrow Aspirate Concentrate Injections for Symptomatic Knee Osteoarthritis. *Stem Cells Transl. Med.* **2019**, *8*, 1149–1156. [CrossRef]
16. Ota, S.; Kurokouchi, K.; Takahashi, S.; Yoda, M.; Yamamoto, R.; Sakai, T. Relationship between patellar mobility and patellofemoral joint cartilage degeneration after anterior cruciate ligament reconstruction. *Nagoya J. Med. Sci.* **2017**, *79*, 487–495. [CrossRef]
17. Bijlsma, J.W.; Berenbaum, F.; Lafeber, F.P. Osteoarthritis: An update with relevance for clinical practice. *Lancet* **2011**, *377*, 2115–2126. [CrossRef]
18. Prieto-Alhambra, D.; Judge, A.; Javaid, M.K.; Cooper, C.; Diez-Perez, A.; Arden, N.K. Incidence and risk factors for clinically diagnosed knee, hip and hand osteoarthritis: Influences of age, gender and osteoarthritis affecting other joints. *Ann. Rheum Dis.* **2014**, *73*, 1659–1664. [CrossRef]
19. Martel-Pelletier, J.; Barr, A.J.; Cicuttini, F.M.; Conaghan, P.G.; Cooper, C.; Goldring, M.B.; Goldring, S.R.; Jones, G.; Teichtahl, A.J.; Pelletier, J.P. Osteoarthritis. *Nat. Rev. Dis. Primers* **2016**, *2*, 16072. [CrossRef]
20. Palazzo, C.; Nguyen, C.; Lefevre-Colau, M.M.; Rannou, F.; Poiraudeau, S. Risk factors and burden of osteoarthritis. *Ann. Phys. Rehabil. Med.* **2016**, *59*, 134–138. [CrossRef]
21. Sato, M.; Uchida, K.; Nakajima, H.; Miyazaki, T.; Guerrero, A.R.; Watanabe, S.; Roberts, S.; Baba, H. Direct transplantation of mesenchymal stem cells into the knee joints of Hartley strain guinea pigs with spontaneous osteoarthritis. *Arthritis Res. Ther.* **2012**, *14*, R31. [CrossRef]
22. Ulivi, M.; Meroni, V.; Viganò, M.; Colombini, A.; Lombardo, M.D.M.; Rossi, N.; Orlandini, L.; Messina, C.; Sconfienza, L.M.; Peretti, G.M.; et al. Micro-fragmented adipose tissue (mFAT) associated with arthroscopic debridement provides functional improvement in knee osteoarthritis: A randomized controlled trial. *Knee Surg. Sports Traumatol. Arthrosc.* **2022**, 1–12. [CrossRef] [PubMed]
23. Polancec, D.; Zenic, L.; Hudetz, D.; Boric, I.; Jelec, Z.; Rod, E.; Vrdoljak, T.; Skelin, A.; Plecko, M.; Turkalj, M.; et al. Immunophenotyping of a Stromal Vascular Fraction from Microfragmented Lipoaspirate Used in Osteoarthritis Cartilage Treatment and Its Lipoaspirate Counterpart. *Genes* **2019**, *10*, 474. [CrossRef] [PubMed]
24. Murphy, J.M.; Dixon, K.; Beck, S.; Fabian, D.; Feldman, A.; Barry, F. Reduced chondrogenic and adipogenic activity of mesenchymal stem cells from patients with advanced osteoarthritis. *Arthritis Rheum.* **2002**, *46*, 704–713. [CrossRef] [PubMed]
25. Murphy, J.M.; Fink, D.J.; Hunziker, E.B.; Barry, F.P. Stem cell therapy in a caprine model of osteoarthritis. *Arthritis Rheum.* **2003**, *48*, 3464–3474. [CrossRef]
26. Zhu, Y.; Liu, T.; Song, K.; Fan, X.; Ma, X.; Cui, Z. Adipose-derived stem cell: A better stem cell than BMSC. *Cell. Biochem. Funct.* **2008**, *26*, 664–675. [CrossRef]

27. Barfod, K.W.; Blønd, L. Treatment of osteoarthritis with autologous and microfragmented adipose tissue. *Dan. Med. J.* **2019**, *66*, A5565.
28. Peeters, C.M.; Leijs, M.J.; Reijman, M.; van Osch, G.J.; Bos, P.K. Safety of intra-articular cell-therapy with culture-expanded stem cells in humans: A systematic literature review. *Osteoarthr. Cartil.* **2013**, *21*, 1465–1473. [CrossRef]
29. Gucciardo, L.; Lories, R.; Ochsenbein-Kölble, N.; Done, E.; Zwijsen, A.; Deprest, J. Fetal mesenchymal stem cells: Isolation, properties and potential use in perinatology and regenerative medicine. *BJOG* **2009**, *116*, 166–172. [CrossRef]
30. Orozco, L.; Munar, A.; Soler, R.; Alberca, M.; Soler, F.; Huguet, M.; Sentís, J.; Sánchez, A.; García-Sancho, J. Treatment of knee osteoarthritis with autologous mesenchymal stem cells: A pilot study. *Transplantation* **2013**, *95*, 1535–1541. [CrossRef]
31. Orozco, L.; Munar, A.; Soler, R.; Alberca, M.; Soler, F.; Huguet, M.; Sentís, J.; Sánchez, A.; García-Sancho, J. Treatment of knee osteoarthritis with autologous mesenchymal stem cells: Two-year follow-up results. *Transplantation* **2014**, *97*, e66–e68. [CrossRef]
32. Davatchi, F.; Sadeghi Abdollahi, B.; Mohyeddin, M.; Nikbin, B. Mesenchymal stem cell therapy for knee osteoarthritis: 5 years follow-up of three patients. *Int. J. Rheum. Dis.* **2016**, *19*, 219–225. [CrossRef]
33. Striano, R.D.; Chen, H.; Bilbool, N.; Azatullah, K.; Hilado, J.; Horan, K. Non-Responsive Knee Pain with Osteoarthritis and Concurrent Meniscal Disease Treated With Autologous Micro-Fragmented Adipose Tissue under Continuous Ultrasound Guidance. *CellR4* **2015**, *3*, e1690.
34. Franceschini, M.; Castellaneta, C.; Mineo, G.V. Injection of autologous micro-fragmented adipose tissue for the treatment of post-traumatic degenerative lesion of knee cartilage: A case report. *CellR4* **2016**, *4*, e1765.
35. Jo, C.H.; Lee, Y.G.; Shin, W.H.; Kim, H.; Chai, J.W.; Jeong, E.C.; Kim, J.E.; Shim, H.; Shin, J.S.; Shin, I.S.; et al. Intra-articular injection of mesenchymal stem cells for the treatment of osteoarthritis of the knee: A proof-of-concept clinical trial. *Stem Cells* **2014**, *32*, 1254–1266. [CrossRef]
36. Sekiya, I.; Muneta, T.; Horie, M.; Koga, H. Arthroscopic Transplantation of Synovial Stem Cells Improves Clinical Outcomes in Knees With Cartilage Defects. *Clin. Orthop. Relat. Res.* **2015**, *473*, 2316–2326. [CrossRef]
37. Vega, A.; Martín-Ferrero, M.A.; Del Canto, F.; Alberca, M.; García, V.; Munar, A.; Orozco, L.; Soler, R.; Fuertes, J.J.; Huguet, M.; et al. Treatment of Knee Osteoarthritis with Allogeneic Bone Marrow Mesenchymal Stem Cells: A Randomized Controlled Trial. *Transplantation* **2015**, *99*, 1681–1690. [CrossRef]
38. Baraliakos, X.; Braun, J.; Conaghan, P.G.; Østergaard, M.; Pincus, T. Update on imaging in rheumatic diseases. *Clin. Exp. Rheumatol.* **2018**, *36* (Suppl. 114), 2.
39. Van Rossom, S.; Wesseling, M.; Van Assche, D.; Jonkers, I. Topographical Variation of Human Femoral Articular Cartilage Thickness, T1rho and T2 Relaxation Times Is Related to Local Loading during Walking. *Cartilage* **2019**, *10*, 229–237. [CrossRef]

Disclaimer/Publisher's Note: The statements, opinions and data contained in all publications are solely those of the individual author(s) and contributor(s) and not of MDPI and/or the editor(s). MDPI and/or the editor(s) disclaim responsibility for any injury to people or property resulting from any ideas, methods, instructions or products referred to in the content.

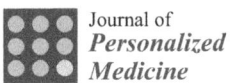

Article

Identification of Immune-Related Risk Genes in Osteoarthritis Based on Bioinformatics Analysis and Machine Learning

Jintao Xu [1], Kai Chen [1], Yaohui Yu [1], Yishu Wang [1], Yi Zhu [1], Xiangjie Zou [2] and Yiqiu Jiang [1,*]

[1] Department of Sports Medicine and Joint Surgery, Nanjing First Hospital, Nanjing Medical University, Nanjing 210000, China
[2] Jiangsu Province Hospital, The First Affiliated Hospital With Nanjing Medical University, Nanjing 210000, China
* Correspondence: jyq_3000@163.com

Abstract: In this research, we aimed to perform a comprehensive bioinformatic analysis of immune cell infiltration in osteoarthritic cartilage and synovium and identify potential risk genes. Datasets were downloaded from the Gene Expression Omnibus database. We integrated the datasets, removed the batch effects and analyzed immune cell infiltration along with differentially expressed genes (DEGs). Weighted gene co-expression network analysis (WGCNA) was used to identify the positively correlated gene modules. LASSO (least absolute shrinkage and selection operator)-cox regression analysis was performed to screen the characteristic genes. The intersection of the DEGs, characteristic genes and module genes was identified as the risk genes. The WGCNA analysis demonstrates that the blue module was highly correlated and statistically significant as well as enriched in immune-related signaling pathways and biological functions in the KEGG and GO enrichment. LASSO-cox regression analysis screened 11 characteristic genes from the hub genes of the blue module. After the DEG, characteristic gene and immune-related gene datasets were intersected, three genes, PTGS1, HLA-DMB and GPR137B, were identified as the risk genes in this research. In this research, we identified three risk genes related to the immune system in osteoarthritis and provide a feasible approach to drug development in the future.

Keywords: WGCNA; osteoarthritis; RNA-seq; disease markers; immune

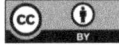

1. Introduction

Osteoarthritis (OA) is a multifactorial disease affecting millions of people worldwide [1]. The gold standard in the clinical management of OA patients is joint replacement surgery in the terminal stage of the disease [2]. Timely intervention is requisite in the early stage of the disease. However, due to the complicated pathogenesis of osteoarthritis [3], there currently is no effective medical treatment except for pain management. Thus, the mechanism of osteoarthritis urgently needs to be clarified.

In recent years, there has been quite some effort in identifying disease markers and predicting the clinical prognosis of osteoarthritis using computational tools. Han et al. first combined WGCNA and immune infiltration in analyzing osteoarthritis-related datasets [4]. Meng et al. made comprehensive use of LASSO regression and SVM-RFE (support vector machine recursive feature elimination) followed by experimental methods and demonstrated the crucial function of PDK1 in regulating the progression of osteoarthritis [5]. Moreover, computational tools also imply a powerful future in terms of predicting disease progression. Janvier etc. reported a new strategy where the progression of knee osteoarthritis could be predicted through assessing the trabecular bone texture in different locations of the knee [6]. Khaled applied use of the Logitboost model in analyzing gray level co-occurrence and local binary patterns to accurately forecast pathological progress [7]. Therefore, computational tools are of great potential in deciphering the secret of osteoarthritis.

The innate immune system has been reported to participate in OA progression [8]. For instance, the macrophages M1 and M2 play different roles in cartilage degradation and regeneration [9]. The T cells secret cytokines and growth factors to impact the extracellular matrix (ECM) [10]. Natural killer (NK) cells exert immunoregulatory effects on the immune response by promoting inflammation [11]. Therefore, it is necessary to determine the expression and distribution of immune cells in osteoarthritis joints.

Synovial lesions contribute to cartilage erosion to a great extent [12]. Immune cells are also significant in synovial inflammation and impact the cartilage through cross-talk [13]. Pro-inflammatory T cells contribute to cartilage matrix degradation from the beginning of the disease [14]. Mast cells can promote inflammation or induce chondrocyte apoptosis in different phases [15]. However, immune cell infiltration differences between the synovium and cartilage have not been studied yet.

In this research, we first combined advanced bioinformatics methods to comprehensively analyze the gene expression and immune cell infiltration in the synovium and cartilage of healthy people and OA patients. Our results for the first time combine datasets from different sources and demonstrate that immune cell infiltration differs significantly in the synovium compared to the cartilage. Collectively, we offer a new strategy in identifying disease markers of osteoarthritis based on focusing prominently on immune-related genes and provide three characteristic genes for future drug development and susceptible population screening.

2. Materials and methods

2.1. Collection of Datasets

We used the keywords "synovium", "osteoarthritis" and "cartilage" to screen the appropriate datasets in the Gene Expression Omnibus database (GEO). Finally, we selected GSE55235, GSE55457 and GSE82107 as the datasets for synovium-related analysis and GSE57128, GSE117999 and GSE169077 for cartilage-related analysis. It should be noted that datasets only involving the groups "healthy" and "osteoarthritis" are rare. Thus, we excluded rheumatoid arthritis samples from a few datasets.

2.2. Merge and Batch Effect Removing of the Datasets

We utilized the R package inSilicoMerging [16] to merge the datasets. The before-merge and after-merge matrix are shown in Supplementary material "Merge Matrix". Furthermore, the empirical Bayes method [17] was used to remove the batch effects. The batch-removed matrix is shown in Supplementary material "Remove_Batch".

2.3. Differentially Expressed Genes (DEGs) Analysis

We utilized the R package Limma [18] to analyze the DEGs. Specifically, we first utilized the lmfit function to find the multiple linear regression of the datasets. Then, we used the eBays function to compute moderated t-statistics, moderated F-statistics, and log-odds of differential expression by the empirical Bayes moderation of the standard errors towards a common value. Finally, we acquired the differential significance of each gene. We set the fold change as 1.5 and the p-value as <0.05 to screen the target genes. The data are shown in Supplementary material "DEGs".

2.4. Immune Cell Infiltration Analysis

To explore the infiltration of immune cells in synovium and cartilage tissues, we utilized the CIBERSORT [19] method in the R package IOBR [20] (a computational tool for immune–oncology biological research) to analyze each sample's 22 different immune cell scores. The correlation analysis was conducted using the Pearson method. We considered $p < 0.05$ as statistically significant. The original data are shown in Supplementary material "Cell infiltration".

2.5. Weighted Gene Coexpression Network Analysis (WGCNA)

We first utilized the expression matrix to calculate each gene's median absolute deviation (MAD) and excluded 50% of the lowest MAD genes. Then, we used the goodSampleGenes method of the R package WGCNA to exclude outlier samples and genes. Subsequently, we constructed a scale-free co-expression network. Furthermore, we merged modules with a distance of less than 0.25. Module eigengene (ME) and gene significance (GS) were used to correlate clinical phenotypes and module genes. We set the MM threshold as 0.8, GS threshold as 0.1 and weight threshold as 0.1 to screen the hub genes.

2.6. Protein-Protein Interaction Network (PPI)

We depicted the PPI network using the online website String. (https://cn.string-db.org/ accessed on 12 November 2022) String is a free online tool that can calculate the network between specified proteins.

2.7. Functional and Pathway Enrichment

We utilized the Kyoto Encyclopedia of Genes and Genomes (KEGG) and gene ontology (GO) enrichment method to analyze the screened genes. For KEGG functional enrichment analysis, we adopted KEGG rest API to acquire the latest gene annotation and for GO functional enrichment analysis, we utilized the gene annotation in the R package org.Hs.eg.db (version 3.1.0). The analysis was performed using the R package clusterProfiler (version 3.14.3). We set the minimum gene set as 5, the maximum gene set as 5000 and considered p value < 0.05 and FDR < 0.25 statistically significant. The results are shown in the bubble diagram.

2.8. Characteristic Gene Screening by LASSO-Cox Regression Analysis

We utilized the R package "glmnet" to perform a regression analysis of the datasets. In this research, we set the survival time as a constant 100, "Healthy" as 0, and "OA" as 1. Thus, we could perform a regression analysis integrating gene expression and OA. The lambda score was 0.027675908746789. The original data are shown in Supplementary material "LASSO-cox".

2.9. Verification of the Targets

We selected the cartilage dataset to perform a correlation analysis between risk genes and OA phenotype-related genes using the Pearson method to verify the reliability of the genes we screened. p value < 0.05 was considered statistically significant.

2.10. Statistical Analysis Software

R software (Austria) was used to calculate the statistical significance.

3. Results

3.1. Intersection of Multiple Datasets

The datasets were obtained from GEO. GSE55235, GSE55457 and GSE82107 provided information for transcriptome sequencing of synovium tissues, while GSE57128, GSE117999 and GSE169077 provided the same for cartilage. The samples were from a healthy population and osteoarthritis patients. We utilized the R package inSilicoMerging [16] to merge the datasets. (Figure 1A,C) As is shown in the box plots and density graphic, the sample distributions of the datasets were quite different. Then, we used the empirical Bayes method [17] to adjust the batch effects of the merged datasets. (Figure 1B, D) This figure indicates that the batch effect was removed effectively. The median was on a line in the box plots, and the mean and variance were close in the density graphic. In conclusion, we successfully merged three independent datasets, thus avoiding the analysis error of using different datasets.

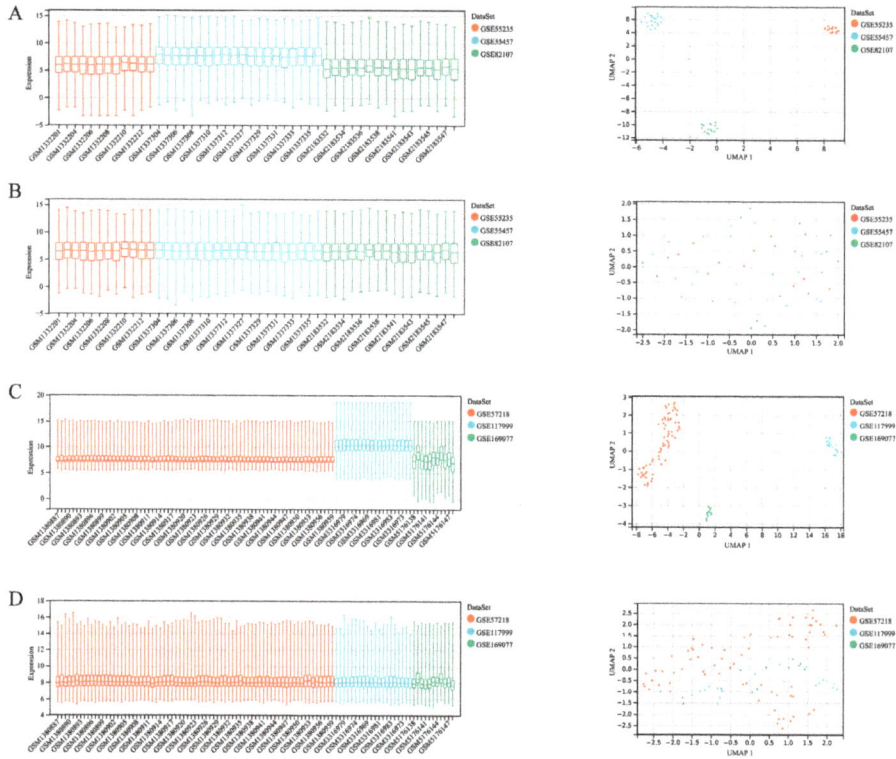

Figure 1. Dataset integration. The results are shown in box plots and density graphics. GSE55235, GSE55457, GSE82107: before merge (**A**), after merge (**B**), GSE57128, GSE117999, GES169077: before merge (**C**), after merge (**D**).

3.2. Differentially Expressed Gene Analysis

Limma is a widely used analytical method to screen differentially expressed genes [18]. We obtained 422 up-regulated genes and 596 down-regulated genes in the synovium dataset (Figure 2A), while 50 up-regulated genes and 11 down-regulated genes were in the cartilage dataset (Figure 2B). The expressions of the top 20 genes are shown in heat maps (Figure 2C,D). These results correspond with the mainstream view that the pathological and functional changes of the articular synovium occur first, even before visible cartilage changes [21]. Thus, we selected the synovium database as the further research object in this research.

3.3. Immune Cell Infiltration Analysis

To explore the function of the immune system in osteoarthritis, we first performed immune cell infiltration analysis using the CIBERSORT method. The results of the stacked bar graphic show that the main infiltrative immune cell in both synovium and cartilage was the M2 macrophage (Figure 3A,C). Noticeably, no statistically significant changes could be observed in the cartilage tissue. However, the infiltration of $\gamma\delta T$ cells, resting mast cells and M0 macrophages increased in osteoarthritis synovium tissues while the infiltration of resting memory $CD4^+$ T cells and activated mast cells was reduced (Figure 3B,D). These results suggest that varying degrees of immune cell infiltration might play a vital role in the pathogenesis of synovial inflammation in osteoarthritis.

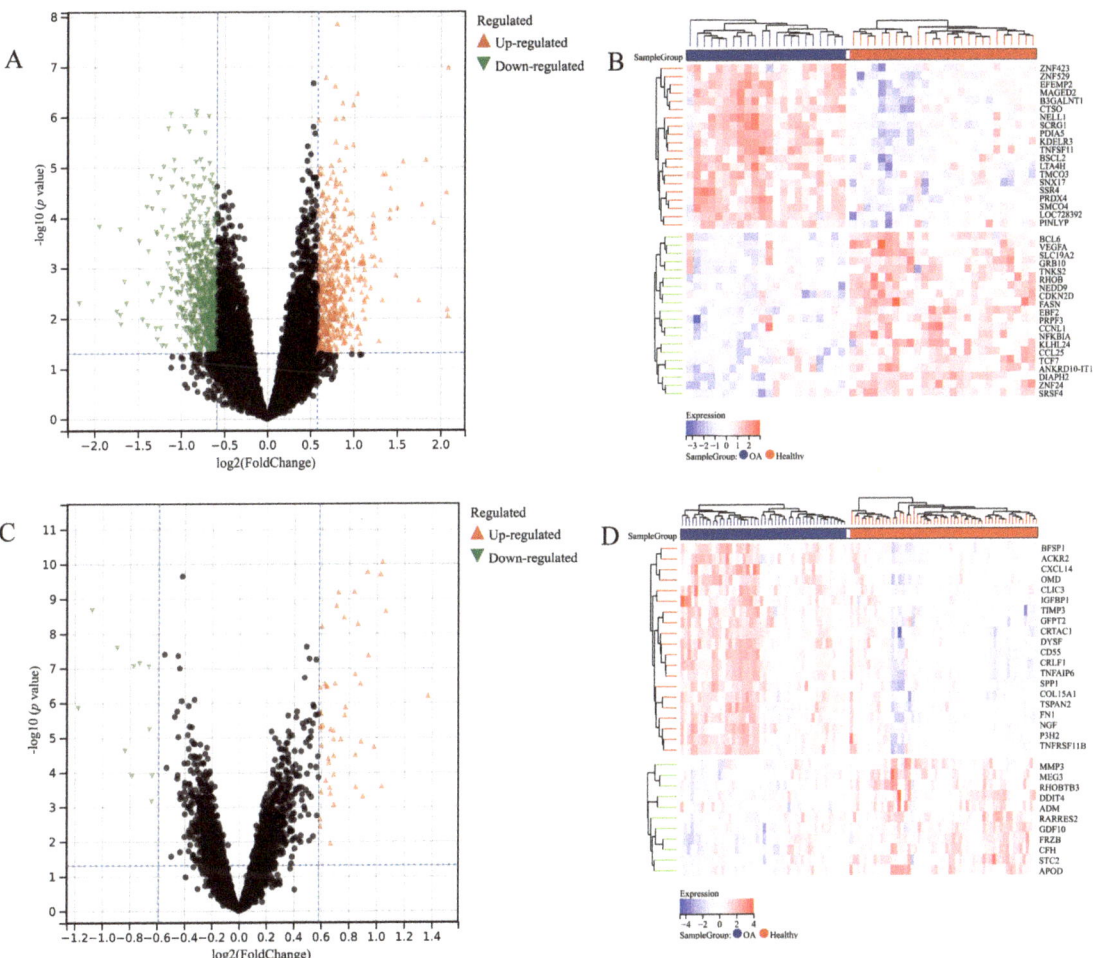

Figure 2. Differentially expressed gene analysis: volcano plot of the synovium dataset, (**A**); heat map of the synovium dataset, (**B**); volcano plot of the cartilage dataset, (**C**); and heat map of the cartilage dataset, (**D**).

3.4. WGCNA Analysis

We obtained 19 co-expressed modules represented by different colors (Figure 4A). Notably, the grey module was considered to not be assigned to any of the modules. The soft threshold was 5, and the scale-free topology model fit degree was 0.86 (Figure 4B). In addition, the average connectivity was 12.26 (Figure 4C). We noticed that light green, blue and light yellow were of statistically significance in all the positive correlated modules (Figure 4D). Based on these findings, we selected these three modules for further KEGG and GO functional enrichment analysis.

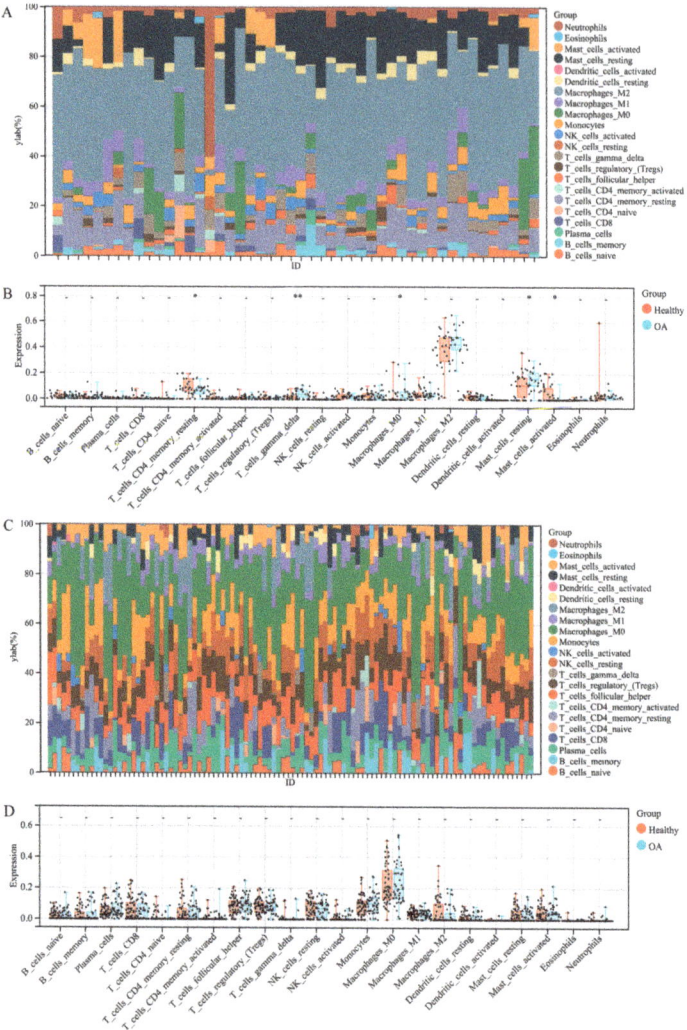

Figure 3. CIBERSORT immune cell infiltration analysis. Stack diagram of immune cells in the synovium dataset, (**A**). Box and scatter plot of the synovium dataset, (**B**). Stack diagram of immune cells in the cartilage dataset, (**C**). Box and scatter plot of the cartilage dataset, (**D**).

3.5. Functional and Pathway Enrichment for the Modules

We performed KEGG enrichment for each module. The light-yellow module is involved mainly in the PI3K-Akt signaling pathway and ECM-receptor interaction (Figure 5A). The enrichment of the blue module consists mainly of human T-cell leukemia virus 1 infection, Th1, Th2, Th17 cell differentiation, B cell receptor signaling pathway, autoimmune thyroid disease and inflammatory bowel disease (Figure 5B), which indicate that the blue module is highly related to the innate immune system. The result of the enrichment of the light green module is of no statistical significance (Figure 5C). Therefore, we selected the blue module as the object of further research. We then performed GO enrichment specific to the blue module (Figure 5D). The functions with the most statistical significance were closely related to the immune system process and immune response. The scatter plot of the blue module exhibited a satisfactory linear correlation between the clinical phenotype and the blue module genes (Figure 5E). We then extracted the hub genes of the blue module and drew a PPI network, which indicated that most of the hub genes interacted with each other (Figure 5F). These results suggest that the blue module is of great potential as the objective module for further characteristic gene identification.

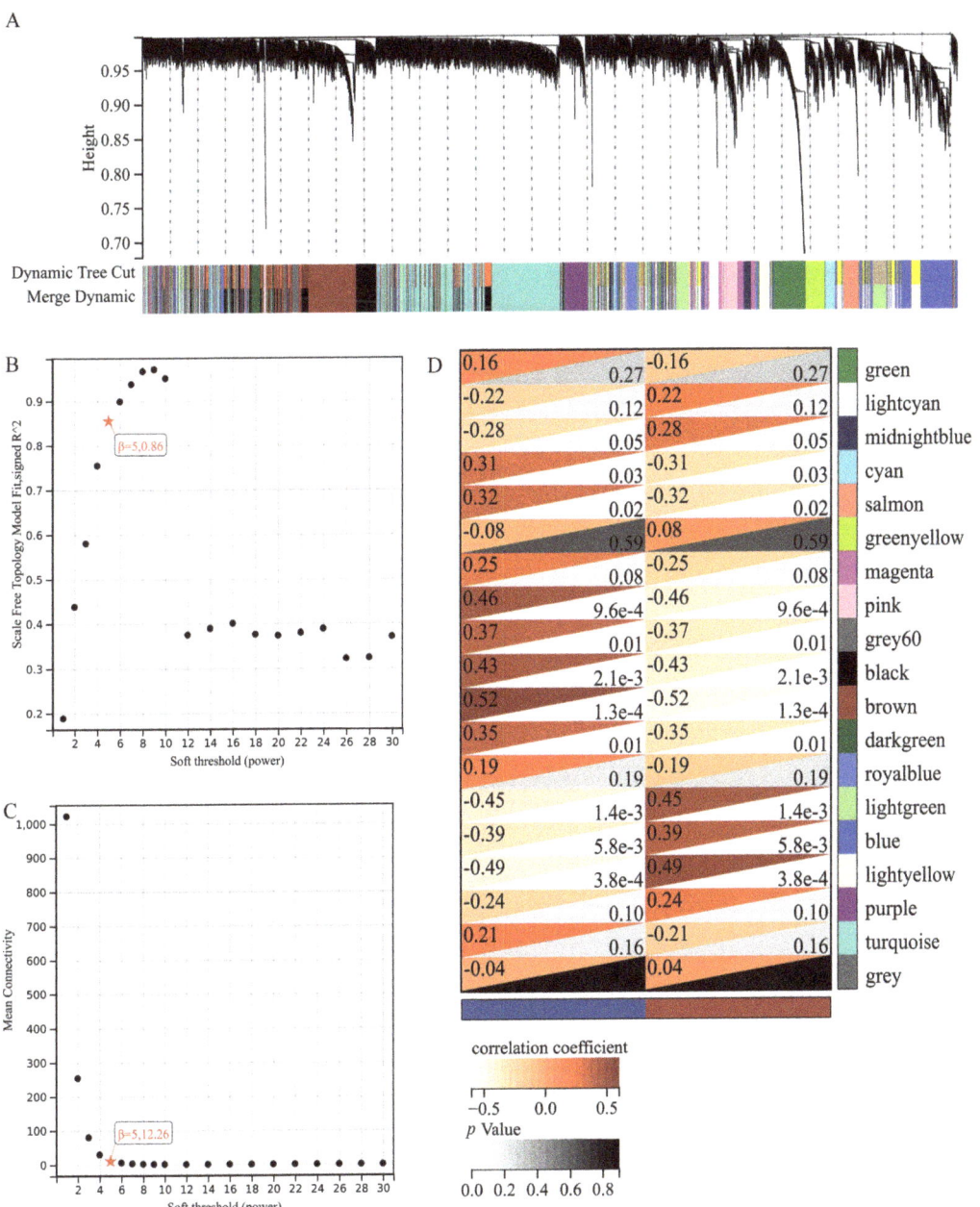

Figure 4. WGCNA cluster detection. Gene cluster (**A**) Independence of scale (**B**) Average connectivity (**C**) Module−phenotype correlation heat map (**D**).

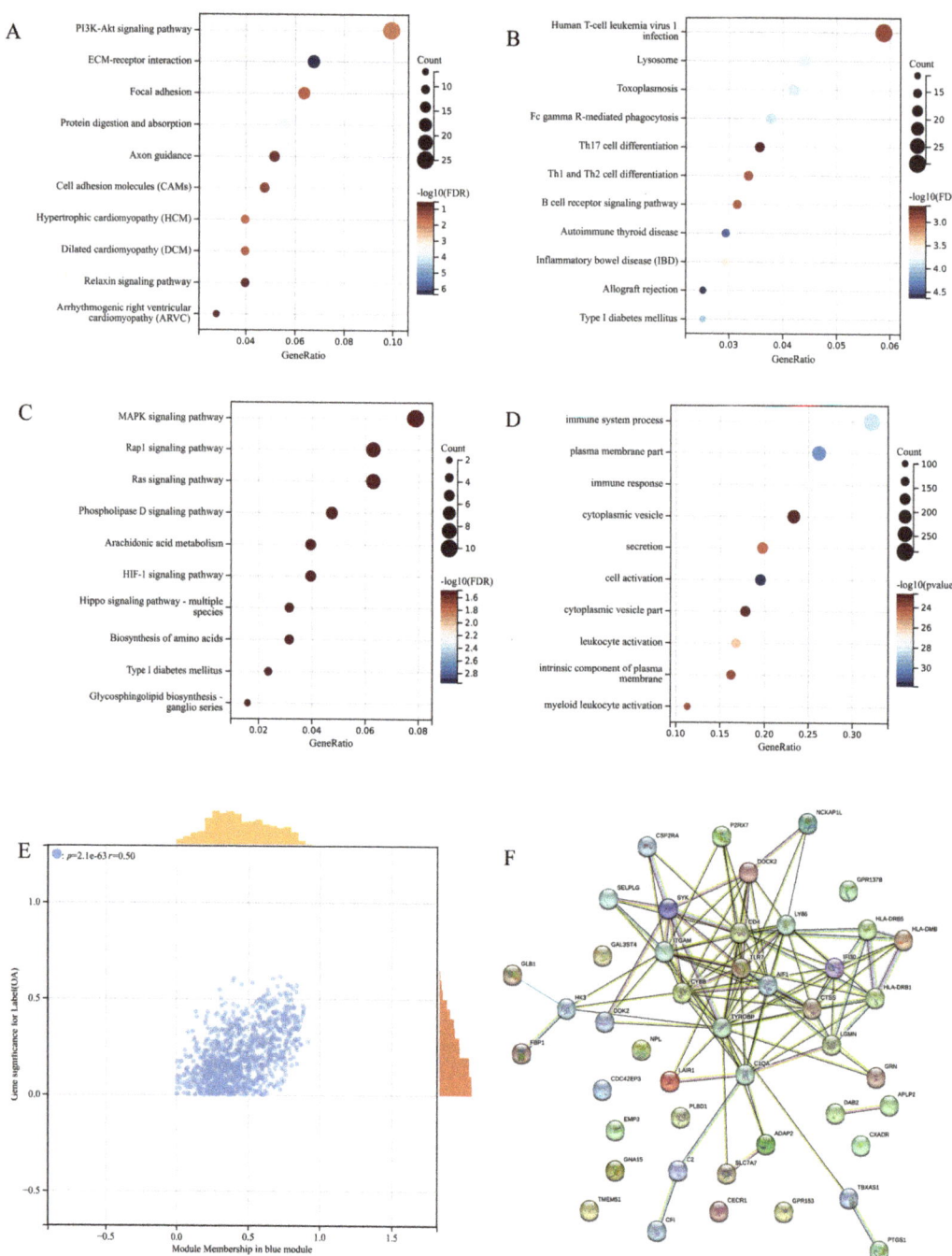

Figure 5. Functional and pathway enrichment and module screen: KEGG enrichment of the light-yellow module (**A**) KEGG enrichment of the blue module (**B**) KEGG enrichment of the light-green module (**C**) GO enrichment of the blue module (**D**) GS−MM correlation scatter plot of the blue module (**E**) PPI network of hub genes (**F**).

3.6. Machine Learning for Prediction of High-Risk Genes

We utilized the LASSO algorithm to identify the characteristic genes of the 39 hub genes (Figure 6A,B). We obtained 14 characteristic genes (shown in Supplementary material "LASSO-cox result") and intersected them with the DEGs and recognized immune-related genes [18]. The final intersection consists of three genes, which are PTGS1, HLA-DMB and GPR137B (Figure 6C). Then, we performed a correlation analysis of the risk genes and recognized genes related to osteoarthritis phenotypes (Figure 6D). Noticeably, the co-expression of MMP13 and these three genes are highly relevant and statistically significant. However, the expression of MMP1 is of no obvious relation with these three genes.

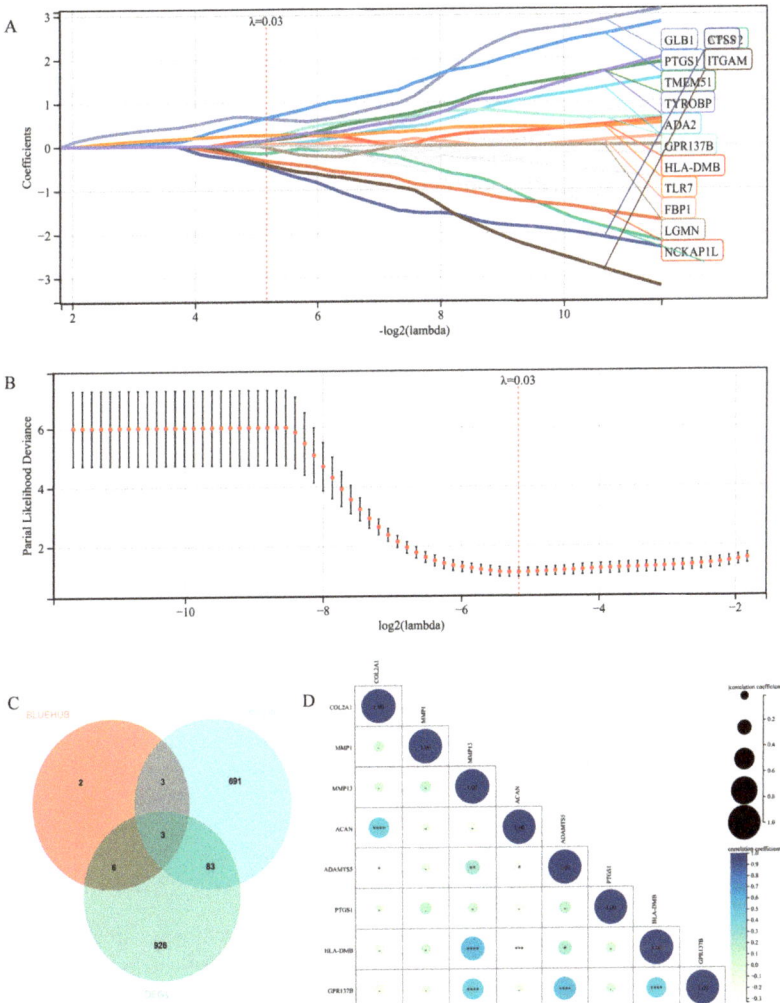

Figure 6. LASSO-cox regression analysis. Coefficient distribution diagram (**A**) Lambda selection (**B**) The intersection of DEGs, immune-related genes and characteristic genes (**C**) Correlation analysis of target genes and OA phenotype-related genes (**D**). * $p < 0.05$, ** $p < 0.01$, *** $p < 0.001$, **** $p < 0.0001$.

4. Discussion

Osteoarthritis (OA) is a disabling disease affecting millions of people worldwide [1]. The factors of OA are manifold and complicated and have not been clarified yet [22]. Extensive low-grade inflammation has been recognized as a critical mediator in the progression of OA [23]. This differs from high-grade inflammation in rheumatic arthritis [24]. Biological therapies that successfully block the inflammation cytokines in RA, such as anti-IL1β, exhibited no promising prospect in the clinical management of OA [25]. Thus, it is urgent to clarify the potential mechanisms of OA to provide new approaches in drug development.

With the rapid development of computer science, advanced bioinformatic analytic methods have been applied in the identification of disease markers and decipherment of pathological mechanisms in osteoarthritis. Since the debut of RNA-sequencing (RNA-seq) technology more than a decade ago [26], it has been an indispensable tool in all kinds of aspects in the genomics field [27]. Differential gene expression (DEG) analysis is the most prominent application of the RNA-seq database [28]. Weighted correlation network analysis (WGCNA) is an R package devised for identifying gene clusters that consists of highly-correlated genes [29]. Based on these clusters, further application of KEGG and GO enrichment analysis allows researchers to focus on the biological function each cluster represents. For interested clusters, a machine learning method-LASSO regression analysis is the optimal option to reduce the dimensionality and screen out the most characteristic genes [30]. The innate system has been recognized to play a vital role in osteoarthritis [8,31]. Consistent activation of pattern-recognition receptors (PRRs) and damage-associated molecular patterns (DAMPs) produces prolonged inflammation [32]. Aging enhances the alterations of the innate system, which is termed "inflamm-aging" [33]. Macrophages and T cells are reported to be the primary immune cell group in the synovium and cartilage [8]. In vivo studies demonstrated that accumulation and activation of macrophages existed widely in OA patients' synovia. The activation of macrophages strongly correlates with osteophytes, joint narrowing and knee pain [34]. However, the specific work pattern of the immune cells remains to be clarified.

Identifying potential disease markers of osteoarthritis has been a research hotspot in different aspects. However, most reports only utilized limited, even single, datasets [35–37]. We believe that merging datasets from different sources could result in a more persuasive conclusion. In this research, we integrated multiple datasets from GEO, which could effectively eliminate the batch difference of studies worldwide. The differentially expressed gene analysis found that the amount of DEGs in synovium outpaces that of cartilage. Under a 1.5-fold change, the amount of DEGs (422 up-regulated genes and 596 down-regulated genes) in the synovium is nearly 20 times as high as the amount in the cartilage (50 up-regulated genes and 11 down-regulated genes).

Then, we performed immune cell infiltration using CIBERSORT bioinformatics analysis to determine whether the immune cells infiltrated differently in tissues from healthy people or OA patients. Unexpectedly, immune cell infiltration in the OA and healthy cartilage exhibited no noticeable difference. Han et al. reported significantly different immune cell infiltration in osteoarthritis, specifically the infiltration of T cells and cytotoxic lymphocytes [4]. We reviewed the datasets selected in the report and found that they not only incorporated the datasets including articular cartilage but also the meniscus. However, we insist that meniscus lesions are a consequence as osteoarthritis develops into its terminal stage [38]. Hence, we suppose that in the research concerning identifying risk factors, it is inappropriate to include the meniscus.

Research targeting immune cell infiltration in the synovium has seldom been reported. What attracted us most was the significant increase in γδT cells in the inflammatory synovium tissues. The γδT cell plays a vital role in the innate immune system [39]; they mainly develop in the thymus and exert major histocompatibility complex (MHC) unrestricted antigen recognition [40]. Activated γδT cells participate in the innate immune process via producing inflammatory mediators [41], which might explain the crucial condition of the inflammation response existing widely in joints with varying degrees of osteoarthritis. Based on these results, we made a reasonable assumption that the immune system might exert its function primarily through the synovial tissues.

Another noteworthy point is that even though the expression of the immune cells in chondrocytes is of no significant difference, the activation of the specific immune cell is difficult to analyze using transcriptome sequencing datasets. We noticed that the macrophage is the prominent cell type in cartilage, and whether it is active in disease progression needs to be researched further. Considering the proinflammatory and anti-inflammatory effects of the different statuses and kinds of macrophages [42], experimental methods are critical concerning these cells.

To explore the correlation between co-expression genes and the clinical phenotype in healthy and OA synovium tissues, we performed WGCNA analysis. In this research, we discuss the gene modules mainly positively correlated with synovial inflammation. The KEGG enrichment of the three most significant modules indicated that the blue module is highly relevant to the immune system. Subsequent GO enrichment also verified this result. We screened the hub genes in the blue module as the candidate risk genes.

The LASSO-cox method was utilized to perform regression analysis to acquire the optimization model [43]. We acquired 11 characteristic genes, ADA2, APLP2, CTSS, FBP1, GLB1, GPR137B, HLA-DMB, ITGAM, LGMN, NCKAP1L, PTGS1, TLR7, TMEM51 and TYROBP. Then, we intersected the DEGs and characteristic genes, recognizing immune-related genes [44]. We finally acquired three risk genes, PTGS1, HLA-DMB and GPR137B. Highly-expressed PTGS1 levels in the synovium promote migration and invasion and inhibit the cell apoptosis of inflammatory synovial cells [45]. HLA-DMB is a prognostic factor in rheumatoid arthritis [46]; however, its role in the processing of osteoarthritis has not been clarified yet. In a genome-wide association study, GPR137B was reported to be correlated with hereditary susceptibility for rheumatoid arthritis [47]. Thus, these three genes could be potential targets in future research on osteoarthritis.

To verify the function of the target genes in osteoarthritis, we performed a matrix correlation analysis of the risk genes and OA phenotype-related genes in the cartilage datasets. Interestingly, the result indicates that the risk genes are highly relevant to MMP13 expression and have remarkable statistical significance. This result is consistent with a theory that chondrocytes probably secrete MMP13 in the cartilage. In addition, the three genes did not correlate with MMP1, which is secreted mainly by synovial cells [48].

This research has a few limitations that have the potential to be research goals in the future. Biological verification must be performed to confirm our results, at least in an animal model. Additionally, we noticed that γδT cell infiltration in the synovial tissue was not researched thoroughly. An establishment of a reliable synovium–cartilage axis model is urgently needed.

Collectively, our research analyzed the immune-related genes in the synovium and cartilage tissues of the healthy population and OA patients. First, we demonstrated that the transformation of immune cell infiltration might mainly exist in the synovium and not the cartilage. These results support the opinion that changes in the synovium might appear before cartilage erosion. In addition, we provided three genes as potential disease markers and future drug development targets.

Supplementary Materials: The following supporting information can be downloaded at: https://www.mdpi.com/article/10.3390/jpm13020367/s1. Supplementary File S1: Merge_Matrix, Remove_Batch, DEGs, cell infiltration and LASSO_cox.

Author Contributions: J.X. and Y.J. provided the idea for this paper. K.C. perfected the analysis details. Y.W., Y.Z. and Y.Y. collected and analyzed the data. J.X. wrote the paper. X.Z. revised the paper. All authors have read and agreed to the published version of the manuscript.

Funding: This research was funded by the National Nature Science Foundation of China (No. 81601954) and the Social Development project of Jiangsu Province (No.BE2020623).

Institutional Review Board Statement: Not applicable.

Informed Consent Statement: Not applicable.

Data Availability Statement: All data presented in this study are available from the corresponding author upon reasonable request.

Acknowledgments: We appreciate the laboratory and equipment provided by Central Laboratory, Nanjing First Hospital.

Conflicts of Interest: This research was conducted without commercial or financial relationships that could be construed as a potential conflict of interest.

References

1. Hunter, D.J.; Bierma-Zeinstra, S. Osteoarthritis. *Lancet* **2019**, *393*, 1745–1759. [CrossRef]
2. Carr, A.J.; Robertsson, O.; Graves, S.; Price, A.J.; Arden, N.K.; Judge, A.; Beard, D.J. Knee replacement. *Lancet* **2012**, *379*, 1331–1340. [CrossRef]
3. Loeser, R.F.; Collins, J.A.; Diekman, B.O. Ageing and the pathogenesis of osteoarthritis. *Nat. Rev. Rheumatol.* **2016**, *12*, 412–420. [CrossRef]
4. Han, Y.; Wu, J.; Gong, Z.; Zhou, Y.; Li, H.; Wang, B.; Qian, Q. Identification and development of a novel 5-gene diagnostic model based on immune infiltration analysis of osteoarthritis. *J. Transl. Med.* **2021**, *19*, 522. [CrossRef]
5. Meng, J.; Du, H.; Lv, H.; Lu, J.; Li, J.; Yao, J. Identification of the osteoarthritis signature gene PDK1 by machine learning and its regulatory mechanisms on chondrocyte autophagy and apoptosis. *Front. Immunol.* **2022**, *13*, 1072526. [CrossRef]
6. Janvier, T.; Jennane, R.; Valery, A.; Harrar, K.; Delplanque, M.; Lelong, C.; Loeuille, D.; Toumi, H.; Lespessailles, E. Subchondral tibial bone texture analysis predicts knee osteoarthritis progression: Data from the Osteoarthritis Initiative: Tibial bone texture & knee OA progression. *Osteoarthr. Cartil.* **2017**, *25*, 259–266.
7. Harrar, K.; Messaoudene, K.; Ammar, M. Combining GLCM with LBP features for knee osteoarthritis prediction: Data from the Osteoarthritis initiative. *ICST Trans. Scalable Inf. Syst.* **2018**, *10*, 171550. [CrossRef]
8. de Lange-Brokaar, B.J.; Ioan-Facsinay, A.; van Osch, G.J.; Zuurmond, A.M.; Schoones, J.; Toes, R.E.; Huizinga, T.W.J.; Kloppenburg, M. Synovial inflammation, immune cells and their cytokines in osteoarthritis: A review. *Osteoarthr. Cartil.* **2012**, *20*, 1484–1499. [CrossRef]
9. Fernandes, T.L.; Gomoll, A.H.; Lattermann, C.; Hernandez, A.J.; Bueno, D.F.; Amano, M.T. Macrophage: A Potential Target on Cartilage Regeneration. *Front. Immunol.* **2020**, *11*, 111. [CrossRef]
10. Ziadlou, R.; Barbero, A.; Martin, I.; Wang, X.; Qin, L.; Alini, M.; Grad, S. Anti-Inflammatory and Chondroprotective Effects of Vanillic Acid and Epimedin C in Human Osteoarthritic Chondrocytes. *Biomolecules* **2020**, *10*, 932. [CrossRef]
11. Benigni, G.; Dimitrova, P.; Antonangeli, F.; Sanseviero, E.; Milanova, V.; Blom, A.; van Lent, P.; Morrone, S.; Santoni, A.; Bernardini, G. CXCR3/CXCL10 Axis Regulates Neutrophil-NK Cell Cross-Talk Determining the Severity of Experimental Osteoarthritis. *J. Immunol.* **2017**, *198*, 2115–2124. [CrossRef]
12. Chou, C.-H.; Jain, V.; Gibson, J.; Attarian, D.E.; Haraden, C.A.; Yohn, C.B.; Laberge, R.-M.; Gregory, S.; Kraus, V.B. Synovial cell cross-talk with cartilage plays a major role in the pathogenesis of osteoarthritis. *Sci. Rep.* **2020**, *10*, 10868. [CrossRef]
13. Manferdini, C.; Paolella, F.; Gabusi, E.; Silvestri, Y.; Gambari, L.; Cattini, L.; Filardo, G.; Fleury-Cappellesso, S.; Lisignoli, G. From osteoarthritic synovium to synovial-derived cells characterization: Synovial macrophages are key effector cells. *Thromb. Haemost.* **2016**, *18*, 83. [CrossRef]
14. Rosshirt, N.; Trauth, R.; Platzer, H.; Tripel, E.; Nees, T.A.; Lorenz, H.-M.; Tretter, T.; Moradi, B. Proinflammatory T cell polarization is already present in patients with early knee osteoarthritis. *Thromb. Haemost.* **2021**, *23*, 3. [CrossRef]
15. Wang, Q.; Lepus, C.M.; Raghu, H.; Reber, L.L.; Tsai, M.M.; Wong, H.H.; von Kaeppler, E.; Lingampalli, N.; Bloom, M.S.; Hu, N.; et al. IgE-mediated mast cell activation promotes inflammation and cartilage destruction in osteoarthritis. *Elife* **2019**, *8*, 39905. [CrossRef]
16. Taminau, J.; Meganck, S.; Lazar, C.; Steenhoff, D.; Coletta, A.; Molter, C.; Duque, R.; De Schaetzen, V.; Solís, D.Y.W.; Bersini, H.; et al. Unlocking the potential of publicly available microarray data using inSilicoDb and inSilicoMerging R/Bioconductor packages. *BMC Bioinform.* **2012**, *13*, 335. [CrossRef]
17. Johnson, W.E.; Li, C.; Rabinovic, A. Adjusting batch effects in microarray expression data using empirical Bayes methods. *Biostatistics* **2007**, *8*, 118–127. [CrossRef]
18. Ritchie, M.E.; Phipson, B.; Wu, D.; Hu, Y.; Law, C.W.; Shi, W.; Smyth, G.K. limma powers differential expression analyses for RNA-sequencing and microarray studies. *Nucleic Acids Res.* **2015**, *43*, e47. [CrossRef]
19. Newman, A.M.; Liu, C.L.; Green, M.R.; Gentles, A.J.; Feng, W.; Xu, Y.; Hoang, C.D.; Diehn, M.; Alizadeh, A.A. Robust enumeration of cell subsets from tissue expression profiles. *Nat. Methods* **2015**, *12*, 453–457. [CrossRef]
20. Zeng, D.; Ye, Z.; Shen, R.; Yu, G.; Wu, J.; Xiong, Y.; Zhou, R.; Qiu, W.; Huang, N.; Sun, L.; et al. IOBR: Multi-Omics Immuno-Oncology Biological Research to Decode Tumor Microenvironment and Signatures. *Front. Immunol.* **2021**, *12*, 687975. [CrossRef]
21. Mathiessen, A.; Conaghan, P.G. Synovitis in osteoarthritis: Current understanding with therapeutic implications. *Arthritis. Res. Ther.* **2017**, *19*, 18. [CrossRef]
22. Krasnokutsky, S.; Attur, M.; Palmer, G.; Samuels, J.; Abramson, S.B. Current concepts in the pathogenesis of osteoarthritis. *Osteoarthr. Cartil.* **2008**, *16*, S1–S3. [CrossRef]
23. Robinson, W.H.; Lepus, C.M.; Wang, Q.; Raghu, H.; Mao, R.; Lindstrom, T.M.; Sokolove, J. Low-grade inflammation as a key mediator of the pathogenesis of osteoarthritis. *Nat. Rev. Rheumatol.* **2016**, *12*, 580–592. [CrossRef]

24. Nettelbladt, E.; Sundblad, L. Protein patterns in synovial fluid and serum in rheumatoid arthritis and osteoarthritis. *Arthritis Rheum.* **1959**, *2*, 144–151. [CrossRef]
25. Chevalier, X.; Eymard, F.; Richette, P. Biologic agents in osteoarthritis: Hopes and disappointments. *Nat. Rev. Rheumatol.* **2013**, *9*, 400–410. [CrossRef]
26. Lister, R.; O'Malley, R.C.; Tonti-Filippini, J.; Gregory, B.D.; Berry, C.C.; Millar, A.H.; Ecker, J.R. Highly Integrated Single-Base Resolution Maps of the Epigenome in Arabidopsis. *Cell* **2008**, *133*, 523–536. [CrossRef]
27. Stark, R.; Grzelak, M.; Hadfield, J. RNA sequencing: The teenage years. *Nat. Rev. Genet.* **2019**, *20*, 631–656. [CrossRef]
28. Conesa, A.; Madrigal, P.; Tarazona, S.; Gomez-Cabrero, D.; Cervera, A.; McPherson, A.; Szczesniak, M.W.; Gaffney, D.J.; Elo, L.L.; Zhang, X.; et al. A survey of best practices for RNA-seq data analysis. *Genome Biol.* **2016**, *17*, 13. [CrossRef]
29. Langfelder, P.; Horvath, S. WGCNA: An R package for weighted correlation network analysis. *BMC Bioinform.* **2008**, *9*, 559. [CrossRef]
30. Guo, C.; Gao, Y.-Y.; Ju, Q.-Q.; Zhang, C.-X.; Gong, M.; Li, Z.-L. The landscape of gene co-expression modules correlating with prognostic genetic abnormalities in AML. *J. Transl. Med.* **2021**, *19*, 228. [CrossRef]
31. Miller, R.J.; Malfait, A.M.; Miller, R.E. The innate immune response as a mediator of osteoarthritis pain. *Osteoarthr. Cartil.* **2020**, *28*, 562–571. [CrossRef]
32. Orlowsky, E.W.; Kraus, V.B. The Role of Innate Immunity in Osteoarthritis: When Our First Line of Defense Goes On the Offensive. *J. Rheumatol.* **2015**, *42*, 363–371. [CrossRef]
33. Franceschi, C.; Capri, M.; Monti, D.; Giunta, S.; Olivieri, F.; Sevini, F.; Panourgia, M.P.; Invidia, L.; Celani, L.; Scurti, M.; et al. Inflammaging and anti-inflammaging: A systemic perspective on aging and longevity emerged from studies in humans. *Mech. Ageing Dev.* **2007**, *128*, 92–105. [CrossRef]
34. Kraus, V.; McDaniel, G.; Huebner, J.; Stabler, T.; Pieper, C.; Shipes, S.; Petry, N.; Low, P.; Shen, J.; McNearney, T.; et al. Direct in vivo evidence of activated macrophages in human osteoarthritis. *Osteoarthr. Cartil.* **2016**, *24*, 1613–1621. [CrossRef]
35. Liang, Y.; Lin, F.; Huang, Y. Identification of Biomarkers Associated with Diagnosis of Osteoarthritis Patients Based on Bioinformatics and Machine Learning. *J. Immunol. Res.* **2022**, *2022*, 5600190. [CrossRef]
36. Liu, H.; Deng, Z.; Yu, B.; Liu, H.; Yang, Z.; Zeng, A.; Fu, M. Identification of SLC3A2 as a Potential Therapeutic Target of Osteoarthritis Involved in Ferroptosis by Integrating Bioinformatics, Clinical Factors and Experiments. *Cells* **2022**, *11*, 3430. [CrossRef]
37. Ge, Y.; Chen, Z.; Fu, Y.; Xiao, X.; Xu, H.; Shan, L.; Tong, P.; Zhou, L. Identification and validation of hub genes of synovial tissue for patients with osteoarthritis and rheumatoid arthritis. *Hereditas* **2021**, *158*, 37. [CrossRef]
38. Englund, M.; Guermazi, A.; Lohmander, S.L. The role of the meniscus in knee osteoarthritis: A cause or consequence? *Radiol. Clin. N. Am.* **2009**, *47*, 703–712. [CrossRef]
39. Wu, D.; Wu, P.; Qiu, F.; Wei, Q.; Huang, J. Human gammadeltaT-cell subsets and their involvement in tumor immunity. *Cell Mol. Immunol.* **2017**, *14*, 245–253. [CrossRef]
40. Song, Y.; Liu, Y.; Teo, H.Y.; Liu, H. Targeting Cytokine Signals to Enhance gammadeltaT Cell-Based Cancer Immunotherapy. *Front. Immunol.* **2022**, *13*, 914839. [CrossRef]
41. Chowdhury, A.C.; Chaurasia, S.; Mishra, S.K.; Aggarwal, A.; Misra, R. IL-17 and IFN-gamma producing NK and gammadelta-T cells are preferentially expanded in synovial fluid of patients with reactive arthritis and undifferentiated spondyloarthritis. *Clin. Immunol.* **2017**, *183*, 207–212. [CrossRef]
42. Zhang, H.; Cai, D.; Bai, X. Macrophages regulate the progression of osteoarthritis. *Osteoarthr. Cartil.* **2020**, *28*, 555–561. [CrossRef]
43. Wang, W.; Liu, W. Integration of gene interaction information into a reweighted Lasso-Cox model for accurate survival prediction. *Bioinformatics* **2020**, *35*, 5405–5414. [CrossRef]
44. Charoentong, P.; Finotello, F.; Angelova, M.; Mayer, C.; Efremova, M.; Rieder, D.; Hackl, H.; Trajanoski, Z. Pan-cancer Immunogenomic Analyses Reveal Genotype-Immunophenotype Relationships and Predictors of Response to Checkpoint Blockade. *Cell Rep.* **2017**, *18*, 248–262. [CrossRef]
45. Wang, C.; Wang, F.; Lin, F.; Duan, X.; Bi, B. Naproxen attenuates osteoarthritis progression through inhibiting the expression of prostaglandinl-endoperoxide synthase 1. *J. Cell. Physiol.* **2019**, *234*, 12771–12785. [CrossRef]
46. Morel, J.; Roch-Bras, F.; Molinari, N.; Sany, J.; Eliaou, J.F.; Combe, B. HLA-DMA*0103 and HLA-DMB*0104 alleles as novel prognostic factors in rheumatoid arthritis. *Ann. Rheum. Dis.* **2004**, *63*, 1581–1586. [CrossRef]
47. Freudenberg, J.; Lee, H.-S.; Han, B.-G.; Shin, H.D.; Kang, Y.M.; Sung, Y.-K.; Shim, S.C.; Choi, C.-B.; Lee, A.T.; Gregersen, P.K.; et al. Genome-wide association study of rheumatoid arthritis in Koreans: Population-specific loci as well as overlap with European susceptibility loci. *Arthritis Rheum.* **2011**, *63*, 884–893. [CrossRef]
48. Burrage, P.S.; Mix, K.S.; Brinckerhoff, C.E. Matrix Metalloproteinases: Role In Arthritis. *Front. Biosci.* **2006**, *11*, 529–543. [CrossRef]

Disclaimer/Publisher's Note: The statements, opinions and data contained in all publications are solely those of the individual author(s) and contributor(s) and not of MDPI and/or the editor(s). MDPI and/or the editor(s) disclaim responsibility for any injury to people or property resulting from any ideas, methods, instructions or products referred to in the content.

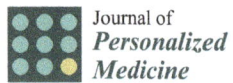 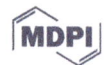

Article

Advancing Osteoporosis Evaluation Procedures: Detailed Computational Analysis of Regional Structural Vulnerabilities in Osteoporotic Bone

Matthew A. Wysocki * and Scott T. Doyle

Department of Pathology and Anatomical Sciences, Jacobs School of Medicine and Biomedical Sciences, University at Buffalo, Buffalo, NY 14260, USA
* Correspondence: mawysock@buffalo.edu

Abstract: Osteoporotic fractures of the femur are associated with poor healing, disability, reduced quality of life, and high mortality rates within 1 year. Moreover, osteoporotic fractures of the femur are still considered to be an unsolved problem in orthopedic surgery. In order to more effectively identify osteoporosis-related fracture risk and develop advanced treatment approaches for femur fractures, it is necessary to acquire a greater understanding of how osteoporosis alters the diaphyseal structure and biomechanical characteristics. The current investigation uses computational analyses to comprehensively examine how femur structure and its associated properties differ between healthy and osteoporotic bones. The results indicate statistically significant differences in multiple geometric properties between healthy femurs and osteoporotic femurs. Additionally, localized disparities in the geometric properties are evident. Overall, this approach will be beneficial in the development of new diagnostic procedures for highly detailed patient-specific detection of fracture risk, for establishing novel injury prevention treatments, and for informing advanced surgical solutions.

Keywords: biomechanics; computational analysis; diagnostic methods; fracture prevention; personalized medicine; patient-specific

Citation: Wysocki, M.A.; Doyle, S.T. Advancing Osteoporosis Evaluation Procedures: Detailed Computational Analysis of Regional Structural Vulnerabilities in Osteoporotic Bone. *J. Pers. Med.* **2023**, *13*, 321. https://doi.org/10.3390/jpm13020321

Academic Editor: Nan Jiang

Received: 7 January 2023
Revised: 6 February 2023
Accepted: 10 February 2023
Published: 13 February 2023

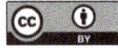

Copyright: © 2023 by the authors. Licensee MDPI, Basel, Switzerland. This article is an open access article distributed under the terms and conditions of the Creative Commons Attribution (CC BY) license (https://creativecommons.org/licenses/by/4.0/).

1. Introduction

Osteoporotic fractures of the femur are a common injury that results in severe health consequences, including high risk of mortality, disability, and dramatically reduced quality of life [1,2]. Much of the previous research has focused on the relationship between osteoporosis and fractures in the proximal femur because this type of fracture is associated with high mortality rates (i.e., 8 percent within 30 days and 25 percent within 12 months) [3–7]. Although proximal femur fractures have been more frequently studied, it is still critical to study diaphyseal and distal femur fractures because they are also associated with high mortality rates. Diaphyseal femur fractures have a 30 day mortality rate of 6 percent and a 12 month mortality rate of 18 percent, and distal femur fractures have a 30 day mortality rate of 5 percent and a 12 month mortality rate of 18 percent [3]. Patients 80 years and older who have diaphyseal femur fractures have a mortality rate of 28 percent within 12 months [8]. Similarly, elderly patients with distal femur fractures have 12 month mortality rates of 30 percent or greater [3,9,10]. Given the high levels of mortality, the high levels of disability, and the considerable burden placed on the healthcare system, it is essential to advance the understanding of how osteoporosis influences the femur's structure [1,9–11].

Aside from the immediate negative consequences of osteoporotic femur fractures, this injury often has very poor patient outcomes regarding healing, restoration of mobility, and restoration of independent living [1,11]. Osteoporosis-associated femur fractures are still considered to be an unsolved problem in orthopedic surgery because it is extremely challenging to acquire effective implant anchorage and because advanced surgical skills are required for administering treatment [9,12]. Clinical research has shown that it is essential for patients to immediately have their mobility restored following osteoporotic bone fractures. However, fracture fixation frequently fails because of the increased fragility of the osteoporotic bone and the decreased structural capacity of osteoporotic bone to securely hold a surgical implant [13].

Individuals afflicted with generalized osteoporosis are at substantial risk of femur fractures, but most fractures of the femur actually occur in individuals who do not exhibit widespread osteoporosis [14,15]. There is evidence to suggest that most fractures of the femur begin within the cortical bone [4,5,16,17]. In particular, results indicate that proximal femur fractures in females often occur due to localized morphological changes caused by osteoporosis [18]. Considering that small structural failures may be the cause of catastrophic fractures, clinically relevant research has shifted to understanding specific aspects of the femur's structure rather than the overall bone density of the femur [19]. However, a more comprehensive understanding of how the process of osteoporosis influences the localized morphological and biomechanical attributes of the rest of the femur is still needed.

Computational analysis of the geometric properties of an osteoporotic femur's structure has the potential to reveal key insights about morphological and biomechanical attributes at specific locations in the femur. The use of the geometric properties from long bones to study biomechanics and functional morphology originated from anthropological studies that employed manual data collection techniques [20]. Over the decades, these underlying principles have been combined with sophisticated digital imaging and 3D modeling techniques to permit improved data collection and data analysis [21,22]. This approach has been used to support the study of the evolution, locomotor capabilities, and behavior of humans as well as other species [23–25]. These computational evaluations have also been used to detect changes in healthy long bones due to distinct habitual loading (i.e., bone functional adaptation) patterns, such as the identification of differences in the lower limb bone characteristics of athletes from various sports [26–29].

In order to more effectively identify osteoporosis-related fracture risk and develop advanced treatment approaches for femur fractures, it is necessary to acquire a greater understanding of how osteoporosis alters the femur's structure and biomechanical characteristics. The current investigation uses computational analyses to comprehensively examine the specific ways in which the femur's structure and its geometric properties differ at specific sites across healthy and osteoporotic femurs. It is hypothesized that healthy and osteoporotic femurs exhibit localized disparities (as opposed to uniform differences across the diaphysis) in their geometric properties.

2. Materials and Methods

2.1. Anatomical Data

We obtained 3D anatomical models of the left femur's osteological structure ($n = 42$) from cadaveric computed tomography (CT) data and used them to calculate the geometric properties. These CT data were made possible by charitable donations to the Anatomical Gift Program of the Jacobs School of Medicine and Biomedical Sciences at the University at Buffalo (UB). The CT data were collected at the Center for Biomedical Imaging of the UB Clinical and Translational Science Institute (CTSI). The UB Anatomical Gift Program and the UB Department of Pathology and Anatomical Sciences approved of the use of these CT data in the current investigation.

This population consisted of both males and females, with an average age of 71.9 years and an age range of 45–92 years. The focus of the current study is the application of a new computational approach to evaluate potential differences in the regional geometric properties of healthy and osteoporotic femurs of humans in general. Given that the skeletal system is subject to changes associated with aging and differences due to sexual dimorphism, a limitation of the current study is that it only assesses osteoporosis in humans overall [30]. Future research is required in order to identify how osteoporosis influences the femur structure in males and females of specific age demographics.

The study consisted of a healthy ($n = 31$) experimental group and an osteoporosis ($n = 11$) experimental group. Several different methods are typically used to assess bone mass for the diagnosis of osteoporosis, and clinicians have been encouraged to diagnose osteoporosis in any older individual that exhibits high fracture risk to help address the underdiagnosis and undertreatment of this disease [31–33]. Most commonly, evaluation of fracture risk is carried out with a bone mineral density (BMD) test using dual-energy X-ray absorptiometry (DXA) in countries where this technology is widely available [34]. BMD tests using DXA were not available for use with the anatomical gifts in the current study. Therefore, osteoporosis was identified using the loss of bone mass in the femur structure extracted from the CT data, which were obtained using uniform Hounsfield units across all specimens with previously established procedures for extracting osteological tissue structure from the CT data [35,36].

The purpose of the current study is to examine the geometric properties of femurs with and without osteoporosis in general. Therefore, rare and unusually advanced cases of severe osteoporosis in which large portions of the femur are entirely absent are beyond the scope of the current investigation and not included within the osteoporosis experimental group. Consequently, the findings regarding the geometric property disparities between healthy and osteoporotic femurs may actually underestimate the morphological and biomechanical consequences of osteoporosis.

2.2. Ethics Approval

This study was performed in accordance with the ethical standards laid out in the 1964 Declaration of Helsinki and its later amendments or comparable ethical standards. The donor cadavers and the associated digital data are the property of the State University of New York at Buffalo. All informed consents were obtained from the donors prior to death by the University at Buffalo's Anatomical Gift Program. Great care was taken in this study to ensure that all potentially identifiable digital cadaver data were removed to make all data anonymous.

2.3. 3D Model Generation

To ensure greater 3D model morphological accuracy and data validity, uniform segmentation was applied to every specimen in the study. This segmentation of osteological structures was carried out using the Kittler–Illingworth (KI) algorithm with robust intensity value thresholding [36–38]. All segmentation was completed using the open-source imaging platform 3D Slicer, and the data were exported as stereolithography (.stl) files [39]. Each of these exported femur structures consisted of both the external structure and the internal medullary cavity structure.

The 3D model optimization was completed using MeshLab, which is open-source 3D mesh processing software [40]. The 3D models were processed using automated functions for isolated piece removal, duplicate face removal, intersecting face removal, T-vertices removal, surface mesh hole closure, and non-manifold edge repair. A consistent mesh complexity of 20,000 triangular faces was used for all specimens in order to attain greater morphological accuracy for the 3D anatomical models [41]. Automated orientation of the 3D models was conducted in order to remove any potential error that would be attributed to rotational and translational differences between the specimens [40].

2.4. Automated Osteological Sampling

The femur specimen's biomechanical length was measured in the publicly available software MeshMixer [42]. The biomechanical length was defined as the average of the measurements between the inferiormost aspect of the superior femoral neck and the distalmost point of medial condyle, as well as between the inferiormost aspect of the superior femoral neck and distalmost point of the lateral condyle, as defined in [43,44]. The y-z plane was defined as sagittal, and the x-z plane was defined as coronal. Automated sampling of each femur was used to obtain 60 evenly spaced cross-sections from the diaphysis ranging from 20 percent (distal) to 80 percent (proximal) of the biomechanical length, which was consistent with previous research [21,45–47].

The 3D anatomical models of the femurs were analyzed in the R programming language and software environment with the alphahull, Rvcg, colorRamps, raster, morphomap, and rgl libraries [21,48–54]. The periosteal and endosteal contours were automatically extracted from each cross-section. In all, 21 semilandmarks were obtained from each contour by sampling with equiangular radii originating from the medullary cavity centroid, which resulted in a total of 1260 semilandmarks per specimen [21]. These mathematically applied semilandmarks were utilized for analysis because diaphyseal bone is an extensive structure that contains very few reliable anatomical landmarks for the comparison of specimens [21,23,55–57].

2.5. Analysis

The cross-sections from each of the 3D models were used to evaluate the morphology of the healthy and pathological femur specimens. The periosteal and endosteal data from the diaphyseal region of the 3D anatomical models were also used to calculate several measurements. Cross-section area measurements were obtained for the total specimen cross-sectional area (i.e., the osteological structure as well as the medullary cavity) and medullary area. Also, the mean bone thickness, minimum bone thickness, and maximum bone thickness were measured at a given cross-section. In addition, periosteal perimeter and endosteal perimeter were calculated from each of the cross-sections.

The cross-sectional data were also used to calculate several parameters that are commonly used to evaluate the biomechanical attributes of osteological structures [23,58,59]. Beam theory, which is an established approach for quantifying long bone biomechanical properties, was applied to the diaphyseal region of the femur [20,28,60,61]. Specifically, the following formulae were utilized in the calculation of the biomechanical data consistent with [21].

The area moment of inertia around the x axis (I_x) for a section was calculated as follows:

$$I_x = \int y^2 dA \tag{1}$$

The area moment of inertia around the y axis (I_y) was defined as

$$I_y = \int x^2 dA \tag{2}$$

In addition, the minimum and maximum moments of inertia were calculated. The minimum area moment of inertia (I_{min}) was determined using the equation

$$I_{min} = \frac{1}{2}(I_x + I_y) - \frac{1}{2}\sqrt{(I_y - I_x)^2 + (4I_{xy})^2} \tag{3}$$

where

$$I_{xy} = \int xy\, dA \tag{4}$$

The calculation of the maximum area moment of inertia (I_{max}) was carried out as follows:

$$I_{max} = \frac{1}{2}(I_x + I_y) + \frac{1}{2}\sqrt{(I_y - I_x)^2 + (4I_{xy})^2} \tag{5}$$

Several section moduli were also calculated for each section. The maximum chord lengths from the x axis and y axis (i.e., d_y and d_x) were used to find the moduli around the x and y axes. The section modulus about the x axis (Z_x) was determined by the formula

$$Z_x = \frac{I_x}{d_y} \tag{6}$$

while the section modulus about the y axis (Z_y) was defined as

$$Z_y = \frac{I_y}{d_x} \tag{7}$$

The minimum section modulus and maximum section modulus were calculated using the maximum chord lengths (i.e., $d_{y\theta}$ and $d_{x\theta}$) from the axes rotated by θ. The minimum section modulus (Z_{min}) was determined with the formula

$$Z_{min} = \frac{I_{min}}{d_{x\theta}} \tag{8}$$

Similarly, the maximum section modulus (Z_{max}) was calculated as follows:

$$Z_{max} = \frac{I_{max}}{d_{y\theta}} \tag{9}$$

Theta (θ), which describes the angle between the principal axis (maximum moment of inertia) or major axis and the x axis (mediolateral axis of the cross section) was calculated with the following equation:

$$\theta = \frac{1}{2} \tan^{-1} \frac{2I_{xy}}{I_y - I_x} \tag{10}$$

The calculation of the polar section modulus (Z_{pol}) was determined using the distance (r) from the centroid to the dA and the formula

$$Z_{pol} = \frac{\int r^2 dA}{r_{max}} \tag{11}$$

The polar moment of inertia (J) was determined with the equation

$$J = \int (x^2 + y^2) dA = \int x^2 dA + \int y^2 dA = I_x + I_y \tag{12}$$

where x is the distance from the y axis, y is the distance from the x axis, and dA refers to the discretized elements of the section.

Additionally, the cortical area (CA), a measurement often utilized as an indicator of the biomechanical properties [24,28,62], was calculated using the cross-section semilandmarks and the formula

$$A = \frac{1}{2} \left| \sum_{i=1}^{n-1} x_i y_{i+1} + x_n y_1 - \sum_{i=1}^{n-1} x_{i+1} y_i - x_1 y_n \right| \tag{13}$$

3. Results

The data differed between the healthy femur experimental group and osteoporosis experimental group for several measurements (Figure S1). The total specimen cross-sectional area data exhibited values for the healthy femur experimental group that were greater than those of the osteoporosis experimental group at all sampling locations (i.e., 80 percent biomechanical length, 60 percent biomechanical length, 40 percent biomechanical length, and 20 percent biomechanical length). Analysis of these total area data revealed that these differences between the healthy experimental group and the osteoporosis experimental group were statistically significant across most of the femur (Table S1). Differences in the medullary area data were statistically significant at the 60 percent biomechanical length and 40 percent biomechanical length sampling locations.

In general, measurements of the bone thickness displayed statistically significant differences between the experimental groups. The mean bone thickness of the healthy experimental group was greater than that of the osteoporosis experimental group at all of the sampling locations along the femur. Similarly, the minimum bone thickness data were greater for the healthy experimental group than for the osteoporosis experimental group at all sampling locations. The maximum bone thickness data were comparable to the mean thickness and minimum thickness data, with greater values occurring for the healthy femurs than for the osteoporotic femurs. These differences in maximum bone thickness were statistically significant at the 80 percent biomechanical length, 60 percent biomechanical length, and 40 percent biomechanical length locations but did not reach the threshold of statistical significance at the 20 percent biomechanical length sampling location.

Although differences in the mean bone thickness were present at all of the sampling locations, the disparities in bone thickness between the healthy femurs and the osteoporotic femurs were not uniform across the diaphysis (Figure S2). Greater differences in mean bone thickness occurred between the 60 percent and 40 percent biomechanical lengths. In addition, the osteoporotic femurs exhibited a disproportionate reduction in bone thickness at the anterior and lateral regions of the distal diaphysis (20–45 percent biomechanical length). Figure 1 shows how the healthy and osteoporotic femurs exhibited different patterns of bone thickness across the femur.

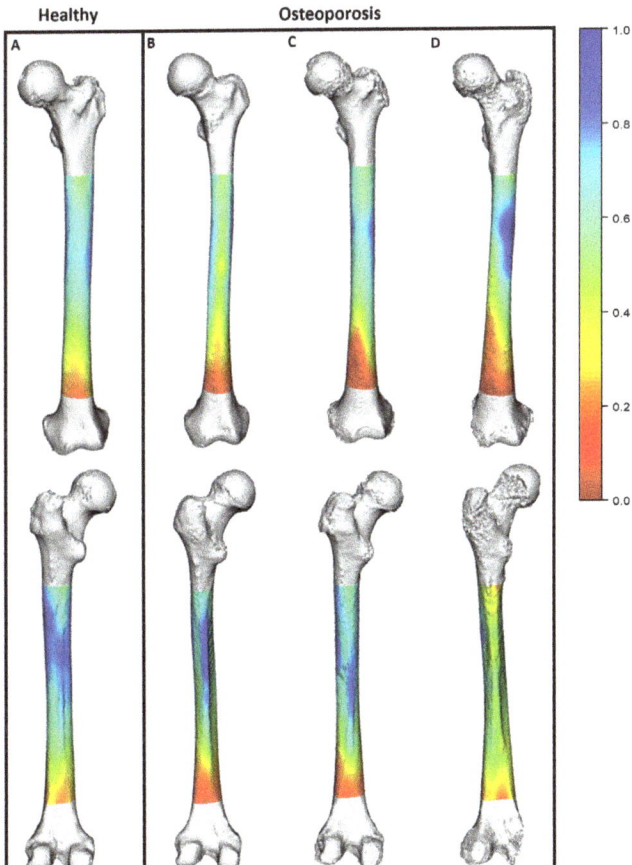

Figure 1. Three-dimensional models exhibiting disparities of morphological data between healthy and osteoporotic femurs. Heat maps show scaled bone thickness data corresponding with each location on the femur. (High thickness depicted in blue, ranging to low thickness shown in red). (**A**) Healthy femur. (**B**–**D**) Three examples of femurs with osteoporosis. Anterior view (above) and posterior view (below) are shown.

The periosteal perimeter data exhibited the greatest consistency between the healthy and osteoporosis experimental groups. No statistically significant differences in the periosteal perimeter were detected at any of the sampling locations along the femur (Figure 2). Alternatively, the endosteal perimeter data had statistically significant differences at the 80 percent biomechanical length, 60 percent biomechanical length, and 40 percent biomechanical length locations (Table S2).

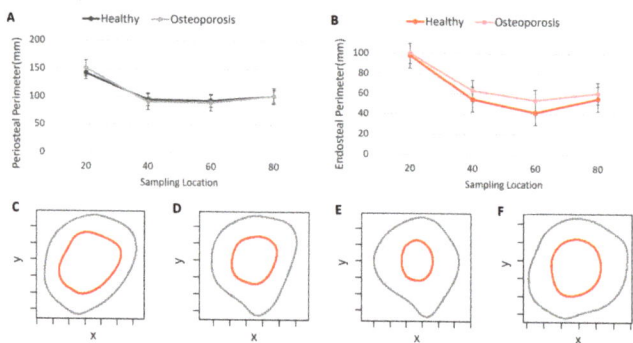

Figure 2. Perimeter data from the healthy and osteoporosis experimental groups. (**A**) Periosteal perimeter data. (**B**) Endosteal perimeter data. (**C**) Periosteal and endosteal perimeters at 80% biomechanical length (BL). (**D**) Periosteal and endosteal perimeters at 60% BL. (**E**) Periosteal and endosteal perimeters at 40% BL. (**F**) Periosteal and endosteal perimeters at 20% BL. Cross-section perimeter examples from a healthy femur.

The area moment of inertia around the x axis and area moment of inertia around the y axis were greater in the healthy femurs than in the osteoporotic femurs at the 80 percent biomechanical length, 60 percent biomechanical length, 40 percent biomechanical length, and 20 percent biomechanical length locations (Figure 3). These differences between the experimental groups were statistically significant at all sampling locations along the femur (Table S3). Additionally, statistically significant differences occurred in the minimum area moment of inertia data and the maximum area moment of inertia data between the healthy experimental group and the osteoporosis experimental group. The average area moment of inertia data of the osteoporosis experimental group had values that were approximately 62–73 percent of those from the healthy experimental group. The greatest difference in all of these measurements was evident at the 20 percent biomechanical length location. At this most distal sampling location, the osteoporotic femur average area moment of inertia around the x axis was only 62 percent of the healthy femur average.

The section modulus about the x axis data as well as the section modulus about the y axis data were greater for the healthy experimental group than for the osteoporosis experimental group, a finding that occurred at all sampling locations (Figure 4). In addition, the minimum section modulus and maximum section modulus values of the healthy experimental group were greater than the corresponding values of the osteoporosis experimental group. These dissimilarities in the data between the experimental groups were statistically significant at all of the sampling locations (Table S4). Overall, the section moduli values of the osteoporosis experimental group were approximately 61–76 percent of those in the healthy experimental group. The largest dissimilarities within each of the section modulus measurements occurred at the 20 percent biomechanical length location. Specifically, the section modulus about the x axis at the 20 percent biomechanical length location was the measurement that had the greatest disparity. The osteoporotic femurs had an average section modulus about the x axis that was merely 61 percent of the average section modulus about the x axis of the healthy femurs.

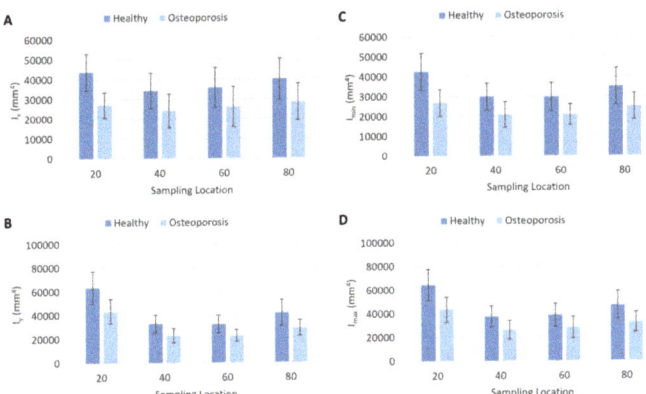

Figure 3. Plots of area moment of inertia data from the healthy and osteoporosis experimental groups. (**A**) Area moment of inertia around the x axis (I_x). (**B**) Area moment of inertia around the y axis (I_y). (**C**) Minimum area moment of inertia (I_{min}). (**D**) Maximum area moment of inertia (I_{max}). Sampling location = percentage of biomechanical length.

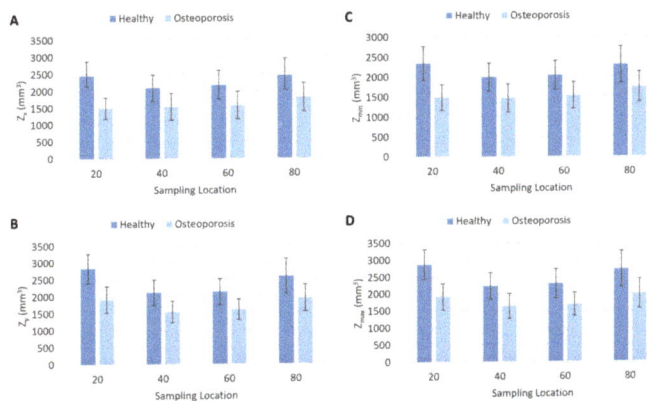

Figure 4. Plots of section modulus data from the healthy and osteoporosis experimental groups. (**A**) Section modulus about the x axis (Z_x). (**B**) Section modulus about the y axis (Z_y). (**C**) Minimum section modulus (Z_{min}). (**D**) Maximum section modulus (Z_{max}). Sampling location = percentage of biomechanical length.

The healthy and osteoporosis experimental groups displayed statistically significant differences in the polar section modulus at sampling locations across the diaphysis (Table S5). At the 80 percent biomechanical length, 60 percent biomechanical length, and 40 percent biomechanical length locations, the osteoporotic femurs had average values that were about 72–74 percent of the corresponding values observed in the healthy femurs (Figure 5). The largest difference in the polar section modulus data occurred at the 20 percent biomechanical length location, where the average value for the osteoporotic femurs was approximately 65 percent of the average value for the healthy femurs. In contrast, the theta values remained consistent between the experimental groups at all sampling locations.

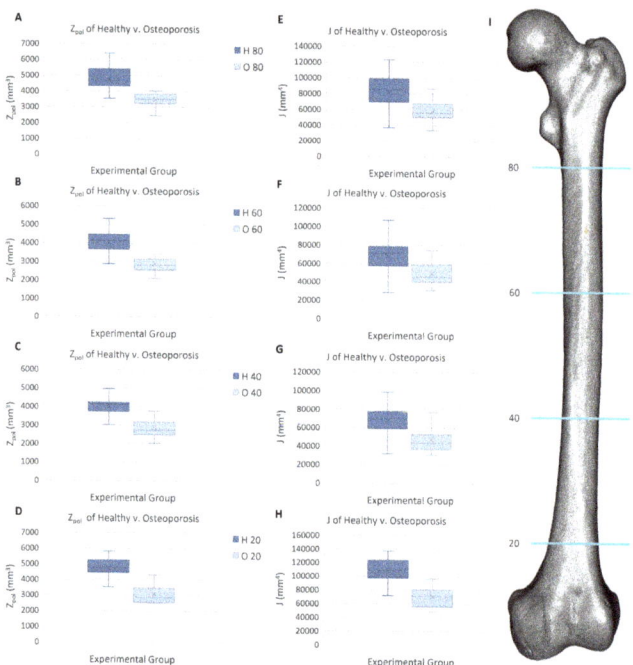

Figure 5. Biomechanical data of the healthy and osteoporosis experimental groups at four sampling locations along the biomechanical length (BL) of the femur. (**A**) Polar section modulus (Z_{pol}) at 80% BL. (**B**) Z_{pol} at 60% BL. (**C**) Z_{pol} at 40% BL. (**D**) Z_{pol} at 20% BL. (**E**) Polar moment of inertia (J) at 80% BL. (**F**) J at 60% BL. (**G**) J at 40% BL. (**H**) J at 20% BL. (**I**) Femur 3D model showing sampling locations (blue).

Akin to the polar section modulus findings, the polar moment of inertia data were significantly different between the healthy and osteoporosis experimental groups. The 80 percent biomechanical length, 60 percent biomechanical length, and 40 percent biomechanical length sampling locations displayed similar variation between the data of the experimental groups, with the osteoporosis experimental group having mean polar moment of inertia values that were approximately 70–72 percent of the healthy experimental group values. A more marked difference occurred at the 20 percent biomechanical length location, where the osteoporotic femurs had a mean value that was about 66 percent of the mean value found for the healthy femurs.

Similar to most of the other quantitative measurements, statistically significant differences in the cortical area data of the healthy and osteoporosis experimental groups were evident at all sampling locations. In all cases, the healthy experimental group had cortical area data that were greater than those of the osteoporosis experimental group (Figure 6). The osteoporotic femurs had a mean cortical area that was approximately 75 percent of the mean cortical area of the healthy femurs at the 80 percent biomechanical length location. Greater differences occurred at the 60 percent biomechanical length, 40 percent biomechanical length, and 20 percent biomechanical length sampling locations. The osteoporotic femurs had cortical areas that were 72 percent, 70 percent, and 70 percent of the cortical areas of the healthy femurs, respectively.

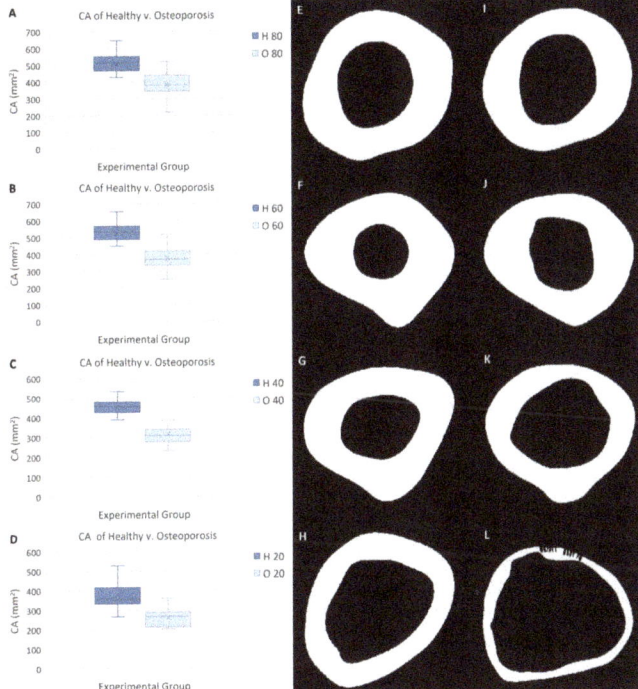

Figure 6. Cortical area (CA) data of healthy and osteoporosis experimental groups. (**A**) CA data from 80% biomechanical length (BL). (**B**) CA from 60% BL. (**C**) CA from 40% BL. (**D**) CA from 20% BL. (**E**) Healthy femur CA (shown in white) at 80% BL. (**F**) Healthy femur CA at 60% BL. (**G**) Healthy femur CA at 40% BL. (**H**) Healthy femur CA at 20% BL. (**I**) Osteoporotic femur CA at 80% BL. (**J**) Osteoporotic femur CA at 60% BL. (**K**) Osteoporotic femur CA at 40% BL. (**L**) Osteoporotic femur CA at 20% BL.

4. Discussion

The current study utilized 3D anatomical models to comprehensively examine the geometric data of healthy femurs and those with osteoporosis. Although these data represent both the morphological attributes and biomechanical attributes of the bones based on beam theory, it is important to note that bone strength is also dependent on the material properties of the specimen being tested [20,28,60,61]. The ongoing study of osteoporosis should continue to examine how variations in the osteological tissue material properties influence the biomechanical performance of various bones overall and at localized regions along bones.

Multiple measurements of morphological data from the healthy femur experimental group were consistent with previous studies that focused on healthy femurs. Specifically, the total area and medullary area data were comparable to those found in prior research [21,63]. Additionally, the healthy femur cortical area, section modulus about the x axis, section modulus about the y axis, and polar section modulus data were similar to those in previous examinations of healthy femurs [24,63].

Statistically significant differences between the healthy femurs and osteoporotic femurs were evident in multiple measurements at several locations across the diaphysis. These results are consistent with previous research, which found that the geometric properties measured from diaphyseal bone are effective for detecting the loss of bone tissue that is due to osteoporosis [58]. In particular, the morphological differences between the femurs of the healthy and osteoporosis experimental groups were especially apparent in the mean bone thickness, minimum bone thickness, and maximum bone thickness, which exhibited statistically significant differences at nearly every sampling location along the femur.

What is more, the data indicate that these differences in femur morphology for the healthy and osteoporosis experimental groups were not uniform across the diaphysis. Compared with the healthy femurs, the osteoporotic femurs had a severely reduced bone thickness at the 40 percent biomechanical length to 60 percent biomechanical length locations, which was further supported by the osteoporotic femurs having significantly greater medullary areas at these sampling locations. Additionally, the results revealed that a disproportionate reduction in mean bone thickness occurred at the anterior and lateral regions of the distal diaphysis in the femurs with osteoporosis. These results for the femoral diaphysis are consistent with previous findings for the femoral neck, which showed localized reductions in cortical bone thickness that were associated with fractures [14].

The geometric properties of the moments of inertia and section moduli are considered to be among the best data for assessing biomechanical capacities [59]. Compared with the healthy femur data, the osteoporotic femur data exhibited the greatest relative decreases in the moments of inertia and section moduli at the 20 percent biomechanical length location. Specifically, the greatest relative differences between the healthy and osteoporotic femurs occurred in the area moment of inertia about the x axis and the section modulus about the x axis. These results demonstrate that the osteoporotic femurs, when compared with the healthy femurs, were proportionately less resistant to bending in the anteroposterior plane at the distal diaphysis (i.e., 20 percent biomechanical length), a finding which suggests that osteoporotic femurs may be particularly vulnerable to fractures in this part of the femur [45,64].

The results also suggest that torsional rigidity is reduced in osteoporotic femurs when compared with healthy femurs. The polar section modulus and the polar moment of inertia data exhibited statistically significant differences at all sampling locations. For each measurement, the greatest disparity between the healthy and osteoporotic femurs was found at the 20 percent biomechanical length location, which suggests that osteoporotic femurs might be particularly less resistant to torsional forces at the distal diaphysis.

The cortical area data, which are indicative of the rigidity or strength of the femur when it comes to axial compression or compressive loading, were also significantly smaller at all sampling locations for the osteoporotic femurs when compared with the healthy femurs [24,28,45,64–68]. Interestingly, unlike other measurements, the cortical area data showed the greatest differences between the healthy and osteoporotic femurs at the 20 percent and 40 percent biomechanical length locations. Therefore, it appears that femurs afflicted with osteoporosis may be more susceptible to compressive fractures in the inferior half of the diaphysis. Intriguingly, these findings are consistent with patient outcomes in which diaphyseal and distal femur fractures exhibit poor healing (i.e., fixation failure typically due to nonunion), in which reoperation is necessary for 13.4 percent and 6.1 percent of patients, respectively [69].

Computational evaluation of osteoporosis may be helpful for reducing the high levels of mortality, the high levels of disability, and the great burden on the healthcare system caused by osteoporosis-associated femur fractures [1,9–11]. Such an approach could use patient CT data to offer comprehensive information about the condition of a patient's bones, including the status of osteoporosis at specific regions along a bone with precise quantitative morphological and biomechanical data from regions of interest (Figure 7). This type of advanced evaluation could offer patient-specific insights about regions of bone that are especially vulnerable to fracturing. This information could be used to inform a variety of advanced preventive treatments.

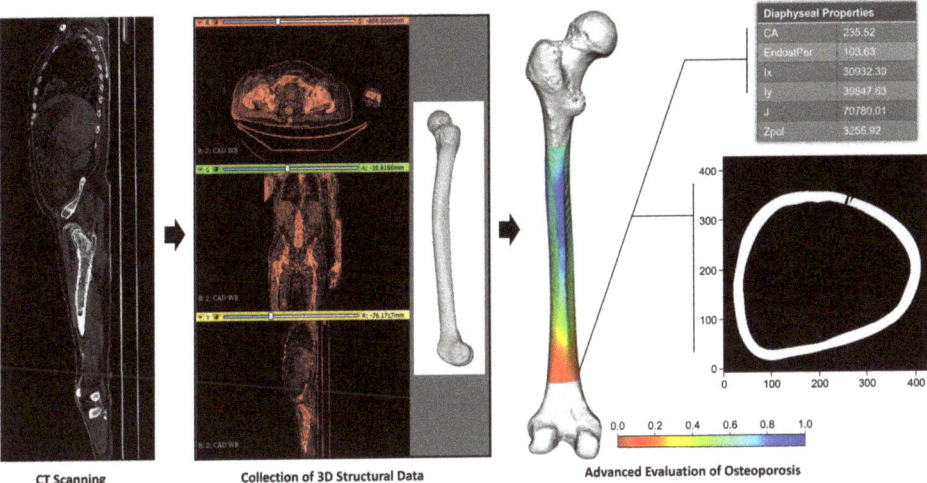

Figure 7. Conceptualization of how CT scans could be used to obtain comprehensive, patient-specific information about osteoporosis risk. Left femur with heat map showing regional bone thickness, a sampling location showing a cross-section of osteoporotic bone, and an example of regional quantitative data that can be calculated at a given sampling location. Cortical area (CA), endosteal perimeter (EndostPer), area moment of inertia around the x axis (I_x), area moment of inertia around the y axis (I_y), polar moment of inertia (J), and polar section modulus (Z_{pol}).

5. Conclusions

Because of the high risk of death associated with femur fractures and the fact that osteoporosis-associated fractures are an unsolved problem in orthopedic surgery, it is essential to fully understand how osteoporosis alters the morphological and biomechanical characteristics of the femur [9,10,12]. The results support the hypothesis that healthy and osteoporotic femurs exhibit localized disparities in their geometric properties rather than uniform differences in these properties across the diaphysis. Furthermore, the results demonstrate that the 3D models obtained from CT scans can be used to identify specific, quantifiable differences in the shape and associated biomechanical properties of osteoporotic femurs. This strategy could be used to improve diagnostic procedures for detecting high fracture risk, to inform novel patient-specific injury prevention treatments, and to develop advanced surgical solutions for treating femur fractures.

Supplementary Materials: The following supporting information can be downloaded at: https://www.mdpi.com/article/10.3390/jpm13020321/s1.

Author Contributions: Conceptualization, M.A.W.; methodology, M.A.W.; formal analysis, M.A.W. and S.T.D.; resources, M.A.W. and S.T.D.; data curation, M.A.W. and S.T.D.; writing—original draft preparation, M.A.W. and S.T.D.; writing—review and editing, M.A.W. and S.T.D.; supervision, M.A.W.; project administration, M.A.W. All authors have read and agreed to the published version of the manuscript.

Funding: This research received no external funding.

Institutional Review Board Statement: Not applicable.

Informed Consent Statement: Not applicable.

Data Availability Statement: The data are contained within the article or Supplementary Materials.

Acknowledgments: The authors would like to thank the anatomical gift donors and their families for advancing this area of medical research. The authors also thank the UB Anatomical Gift Program and the UB Clinical and Translational Science Institute for providing the CT data. In addition, the authors wish to thank two anonymous reviewers for their helpful comments, which improved this manuscript.

Conflicts of Interest: The authors declare no conflict of interest.

Abbreviations

The following abbreviations are used in this manuscript:

CT	Computed tomography
UB	Universtity at Buffalo
CTSI	Clinical and Translational Science Institute
KI	Kittler–Illingworth
I_x	Area moment of inertia around the x axis
I_y	Area moment of inertia around the y axis
I_{min}	Minimum area moment of inertia
I_{max}	Maximum area moment of inertia
Z_x	Section modulus about the x axis
Z_y	Section modulus about the y axis
Z_{min}	Minimum section modulus
Z_{max}	Maximum section modulus
θ	Theta
Z_{pol}	Polar section modulus
J	Polar moment of inertia
CA	Cortical area
BL	Biomechanical length

References

1. Caliri, A.; De Filippis, L.; Bagnato, G.; Bagnato, G. Osteoporotic fractures: Mortality and quality of life. *Panminerva Med.* **2007**, *49*, 21. [PubMed]
2. Glinkowski, W.; Narloch, J.; Krasuski, K.; Śliwczyński, A. The increase of osteoporotic hip fractures and associated one-year mortality in Poland: 2008–2015. *J. Clin. Med.* **2019**, *8*, 1487. [CrossRef] [PubMed]
3. Bergh, C.; Möller, M.; Ekelund, J.; Brisby, H. 30-day and 1-year mortality after skeletal fractures: A register study of 295,713 fractures at different locations. *Acta Orthop.* **2021**, *92*, 739–745. [CrossRef] [PubMed]
4. Carpenter, R.D.; Beaupré, G.S.; Lang, T.F.; Orwoll, E.S.; Carter, D.R. New QCT analysis approach shows the importance of fall orientation on femoral neck strength. *J. Bone Miner. Res.* **2005**, *20*, 1533–1542. [CrossRef]
5. Mayhew, P.M.; Thomas, C.D.; Clement, J.G.; Loveridge, N.; Beck, T.J.; Bonfield, W.; Burgoyne, C.J.; Reeve, J. Relation between age, femoral neck cortical stability, and hip fracture risk. *Lancet* **2005**, *366*, 129–135. [CrossRef]
6. Lotz, J.; Cheal, E.; Hayes, W. Stress distributions within the proximal femur during gait and falls: Implications for osteoporotic fracture. *Osteoporos. Int.* **1995**, *5*, 252–261. [CrossRef]
7. Sollmann, N.; Löffler, M.T.; Kronthaler, S.; Böhm, C.; Dieckmeyer, M.; Ruschke, S.; Kirschke, J.S.; Carballido-Gamio, J.; Karampinos, D.C.; Krug, R.; et al. MRI-based quantitative osteoporosis imaging at the spine and femur. *J. Magn. Reson. Imaging* **2021**, *54*, 12–35. [CrossRef]
8. Bergh, C.; Möller, M.; Ekelund, J.; Brisby, H. Mortality after sustaining skeletal fractures in relation to age. *J. Clin. Med.* **2022**, *11*, 2313. [CrossRef]
9. Canton, G.; Giraldi, G.; Dussi, M.; Ratti, C.; Murena, L. Osteoporotic distal femur fractures in the elderly: Peculiarities and treatment strategies. *Acta Biomed.* **2019**, *90*, 25.
10. Larsen, P.; Ceccotti, A.A.; Elsoe, R. High mortality following distal femur fractures: A cohort study including three hundred and two distal femur fractures. *Int. Orthop.* **2020**, *44*, 173–177. [CrossRef]
11. Kammerlander, C.; Riedmüller, P.; Gosch, M.; Zegg, M.; Kammerlander-Knauer, U.; Schmid, R.; Roth, T. Functional outcome and mortality in geriatric distal femoral fractures. *Injury* **2012**, *43*, 1096–1101. [CrossRef]
12. Kim, J.; Kang, S.B.; Nam, K.; Rhee, S.H.; Won, J.W.; Han, H.S. Retrograde intramedullary nailing for distal femur fracture with osteoporosis. *Clin. Orthop. Surg.* **2012**, *4*, 307–312. [CrossRef]
13. Hollensteiner, M.; Sandriesser, S.; Bliven, E.; von Rüden, C.; Augat, P. Biomechanics of osteoporotic fracture fixation. *Curr. Osteoporos. Rep.* **2019**, *17*, 363–374. [CrossRef]
14. Poole, K.E.; Treece, G.M.; Mayhew, P.M.; Vaculík, J.; Dungl, P.; Horák, M.; Štěpán, J.J.; Gee, A.H. Cortical thickness mapping to identify focal osteoporosis in patients with hip fracture. *PLoS ONE* **2012**, *7*, e38466. [CrossRef]
15. Wainwright, S.A.; Marshall, L.M.; Ensrud, K.E.; Cauley, J.A.; Black, D.M.; Hillier, T.A.; Hochberg, M.C.; Vogt, M.T.; Orwoll, E.S.; Study of Osteoporotic Fractures Research Group. Hip fracture in women without osteoporosis. *J. Clin. Endocrinol. Metab.* **2005**, *90*, 2787–2793. [CrossRef]

16. Treece, G.M.; Poole, K.E.; Gee, A.H. Imaging the femoral cortex: Thickness, density and mass from clinical CT. *Med. Image Anal.* **2012**, *16*, 952–965. [CrossRef]
17. De Bakker, P.M.; Manske, S.L.; Ebacher, V.; Oxland, T.R.; Cripton, P.A.; Guy, P. During sideways falls proximal femur fractures initiate in the superolateral cortex: Evidence from high-speed video of simulated fractures. *J. Biomech.* **2009**, *42*, 1917–1925. [CrossRef]
18. Poole, K.E.; Skingle, L.; Gee, A.H.; Turmezei, T.D.; Johannesdottir, F.; Blesic, K.; Rose, C.; Vindlacheruvu, M.; Donell, S.; Vaculik, J.; et al. Focal osteoporosis defects play a key role in hip fracture. *Bone* **2017**, *94*, 124–134. [CrossRef]
19. Poole, K.E.; Treece, G.M.; Gee, A.H.; Brown, J.P.; McClung, M.R.; Wang, A.; Libanati, C. Response to: Comment on:"Denosumab rapidly increases cortical bone in key locations of the femur: A 3D bone mapping study in women with osteoporosis". *J. Bone Miner. Res.* **2015**, *30*, 1939–1940. [CrossRef]
20. Endo, B.; Takahashi, H. Various methods for measuring the geometrical properties of the long bone cross section with respect to mechanics. *J. Anthropol. Soc. Jpn.* **1982**, *90*, 1–16. [CrossRef]
21. Profico, A.; Bondioli, L.; Raia, P.; O'Higgins, P.; Marchi, D. morphomap: An R package for long bone landmarking, cortical thickness, and cross-sectional geometry mapping. *Am. J. Phys. Anthropol.* **2021**, *174*, 129–139. [CrossRef] [PubMed]
22. Doube, M.; Kłosowski, M.M.; Arganda-Carreras, I.; Cordelières, F.P.; Dougherty, R.P.; Jackson, J.S.; Schmid, B.; Hutchinson, J.R.; Shefelbine, S.J. BoneJ: Free and extensible bone image analysis in ImageJ. *Bone* **2010**, *47*, 1076–1079. [CrossRef] [PubMed]
23. Morimoto, N.; De León, M.S.P.; Zollikofer, C.P. Exploring femoral diaphyseal shape variation in wild and captive chimpanzees by means of morphometric mapping: A test of Wolff's law. *Anat. Rec.* **2011**, *294*, 589–609. [CrossRef] [PubMed]
24. Puymerail, L. The functionally-related signatures characterizing the endostructural organisation of the femoral shaft in modern humans and chimpanzee. *C. R. Palevol* **2013**, *12*, 223–231. [CrossRef]
25. Kivell, T.L.; Davenport, R.; Hublin, J.J.; Thackeray, J.F.; Skinner, M.M. Trabecular architecture and joint loading of the proximal humerus in extant hominoids, Ateles, and Australopithecus africanus. *Am. J. Phys. Anthropol.* **2018**, *167*, 348–365. [CrossRef]
26. Wallace, J.M.; Rajachar, R.M.; Allen, M.R.; Bloomfield, S.A.; Robey, P.G.; Young, M.F.; Kohn, D.H. Exercise-induced changes in the cortical bone of growing mice are bone-and gender-specific. *Bone* **2007**, *40*, 1120–1127. [CrossRef]
27. Carlson, K.J.; Judex, S. Increased non-linear locomotion alters diaphyseal bone shape. *J. Exp. Biol.* **2007**, *210*, 3117–3125. [CrossRef]
28. Shaw, C.N.; Stock, J.T. Intensity, repetitiveness, and directionality of habitual adolescent mobility patterns influence the tibial diaphysis morphology of athletes. *Am. J. Phys. Anthropol.* **2009**, *140*, 149–159. [CrossRef]
29. Niinimäki, S.; Narra, N.; Härkönen, L.; Abe, S.; Nikander, R.; Hyttinen, J.; Knüsel, C.; Sievänen, H. The relationship between loading history and proximal femoral diaphysis cross-sectional geometry. *Am. J. Hum.* **2017**, *29*, e22965. [CrossRef]
30. Jepsen, K.J.; Bigelow, E.M.; Schlecht, S.H. Women build long bones with less cortical mass relative to body size and bone size compared with men. *Clin. Orthop. Relat. Res.* **2015**, *473*, 2530–2539. [CrossRef]
31. Wark, J.D. Osteoporosis: A global perspective. *Bull. World Health Organ.* **1999**, *77*, 424.
32. Siris, E.; Boonen, S.; Mitchell, P.; Bilezikian, J.; Silverman, S. What's in a name? What constitutes the clinical diagnosis of osteoporosis? *Osteoporos. Int.* **2012**, *23*, 2093–2097. [CrossRef]
33. Siris, E.; Adler, R.; Bilezikian, J.; Bolognese, M.; Dawson-Hughes, B.; Favus, M.; Harris, S.; Jan de Beur, S.; Khosla, S.; Lane, N.; et al. The clinical diagnosis of osteoporosis: A position statement from the National Bone Health Alliance Working Group. *Osteoporos. Int.* **2014**, *25*, 1439–1443. [CrossRef]
34. Johnell, O.; Kanis, J.A.; Oden, A.; Johansson, H.; De Laet, C.; Delmas, P.; Eisman, J.A.; Fujiwara, S.; Kroger, H.; Mellstrom, D.; et al. Predictive value of BMD for hip and other fractures. *J. Bone Miner. Res.* **2005**, *20*, 1185–1194. [CrossRef]
35. Lepor, H. *Prostatic Diseases*; W.B. Saunders Company: Philadelphia, PA, USA, 2000; p. 966.
36. Wysocki, M.A.; Doyle, S. The impact of CT-data segmentation variation on the morphology of osteological structure. *Proc. SPIE Med. Imag.* **2021**, *11595*. [CrossRef]
37. Kittler, J.; Illingworth, J. Minimum error thresholding. *Pattern Recognit.* **1986**, *19*, 41–47. [CrossRef]
38. Wysocki, M.A.; Doyle, S. Enhancing biomedical data validity with standardized segmentation finite element analysis. *Sci. Rep.* **2022**, *12*, 1–9. [CrossRef]
39. Fedorov, A.; Beichel, R.; Kalpathy-Cramer, J.; Finet, J.; Fillion-Robin, J.C.; Pujol, S.; Bauer, C.; Jennings, D.; Fennessy, F.; Sonka, M.; et al. 3D Slicer as an image computing platform for the Quantitative Imaging Network. *Magn. Reson. Imaging* **2012**, *30*, 1323–1341. [CrossRef]
40. Cignoni, P.; Callieri, M.; Corsini, M.; Dellepiane, M.; Ganovelli, F.; Ranzuglia, G. Meshlab: An open-source mesh processing tool. In Proceedings of the Eurographics Italian Chapter Conference, Salerno, Italy, 2–4 July 2008; Volume 2008, pp. 129–136.
41. Wysocki, M.A.; Doyle, S. Optimization of decimation protocols for advancing the validity of 3D model data. *Proc. SPIE Med. Imag.* **2022**, *12031*. [CrossRef]
42. Inc., A. Meshmixer. Version 3.5.474. 2017. Available online: www.meshmixer.com (accessed on 1 July 2021).
43. Trinkaus, E.; Churchill, S.E.; Ruff, C.B.; Vandermeersch, B. Long bone shaft robusticity and body proportions of the Saint-Césaire 1 Châtelperronian Neanderthal. *J. Archaeol. Sci.* **1999**, *26*, 753–773. [CrossRef]
44. White, T.D.; Black, M.T.; Folkens, P.A. *Human Osteology*; Academic Press: Cambridge, MA, USA, 2011.
45. Ruff, C.B. Long bone articular and diaphyseal structure in Old World monkeys and apes. I: Locomotor effects. *Am. J. Phys. Anthropol.* **2002**, *119*, 305–342. [CrossRef] [PubMed]

46. Marchi, D. The cross-sectional geometry of the hand and foot bones of the Hominoidea and its relationship to locomotor behavior. *J. Hum. Evol.* **2005**, *49*, 743–761. [CrossRef] [PubMed]
47. Marchi, D. Relative strength of the tibia and fibula and locomotor behavior in hominoids. *J. Hum. Evol.* **2007**, *53*, 647–655. [CrossRef] [PubMed]
48. Rodríguez Casal, A.; Pateiro López, B. Generalizing the convex hull of a sample: The R package alphahull. *J. Stat. Softw.* **2010**, *34*, 1–28. [CrossRef]
49. Schlager, S.; Schlager, M.S. Package 'Rvcg'; R Package. 2014. Available online: https://cran.microsoft.com/snapshot/2014-12-24/web/packages/Rvcg/Rvcg.pdf (accessed on 6 February 2023).
50. Schlager, S. Morpho and Rvcg–Shape Analysis in R: R-Packages for Geometric Morphometrics, Shape Analysis and Surface Manipulations. In *Statistical Shape and Deformation Analysis*; Academic press: Cambridge, MA, USA, 2017; pp. 217–256.
51. Keitt, T.H. Coherent ecological dynamics induced by large-scale disturbance. *Nature* **2008**, *454*, 331–334. [CrossRef]
52. Hijmans, R.J.; Van Etten, J.; Cheng, J.; Mattiuzzi, M.; Sumner, M.; Greenberg, J.A.; Lamigueiro, O.P.; Bevan, A.; Racine, E.B.; Shortridge, A.; et al. Package 'Raster'. R Package. 2015, p. 734. Available online: https://cran.r-project.org/web/packages/raster/raster.pdf (accessed on 6 February 2023).
53. Team, R.C. *R: A Language and Environment for Statistical Computing*; R Foundation for Statistical Computing: Vienna, Austria, 2020.
54. Murdoch, D.; Adler, D.; Nenadic, O. Package 'rgl'. R Package. 2023. Available online: https://cran.r-project.org/web/packages/rgl/rgl.pdf (accessed on 6 February 2023).
55. Gunz, P.; Mitteroecker, P.; Bookstein, F.L. Semilandmarks in three dimensions. In *Modern Morphometrics in Physical Anthropology*; Kluwer Academic / Plenum Publishers: New York, NY, USA, 2005; pp. 73–98.
56. Frelat, M.A.; Katina, S.; Weber, G.W.; Bookstein, F.L. A novel geometric morphometric approach to the study of long bone shape variation. *Am. J. Phys. Anthropol.* **2012**, *149*, 628–638. [CrossRef]
57. Morimoto, N.; Nakatsukasa, M.; de León, M.S.P.; Zollikofer, C.P. Femoral ontogeny in humans and great apes and its implications for their last common ancestor. *Sci. Rep.* **2018**, *8*, 1–11. [CrossRef]
58. Garn, S.M.; Poznanski, A.K.; Nagy, J.M. Bone measurement in the differential diagnosis of osteopenia and osteoporosis. *Radiology* **1971**, *100*, 509–518. [CrossRef]
59. Ruff, C.; Holt, B.; Trinkaus, E. Who's afraid of the big bad Wolff?:"Wolff's law" and bone functional adaptation. *Am. J. Phys. Anthropol.* **2006**, *129*, 484–498. [CrossRef]
60. Ruff, C.B.; Trinkaus, E.; Walker, A.; Larsen, C.S. Postcranial robusticity in Homo. I: Temporal trends and mechanical interpretation. *Am. J. Phys. Anthropol.* **1993**, *91*, 21–53. [CrossRef]
61. Stock, J.; Pfeiffer, S. Linking structural variability in long bone diaphyses to habitual behaviors: Foragers from the southern African Later Stone Age and the Andaman Islands. *Am. J. Phys. Anthropol.* **2001**, *115*, 337–348. [CrossRef]
62. Trinkaus, E.; Ruff, C.B. Femoral and tibial diaphyseal cross-sectional geometry in Pleistocene Homo. *PaleoAnthropology* **2012**, *2012*, 13–62.
63. Lacoste Jeanson, A.; Santos, F.; Dupej, J.; Veleminska, J.; Bruzek, J. Sex-specific functional adaptation of the femoral diaphysis to body composition. *Am. J. Hum. Biol.* **2018**, *30*, e23123. [CrossRef]
64. Lacoste Jeanson, A.; Santos, F.; Villa, C.; Banner, J.; Bruzek, J. Architecture of the femoral and tibial diaphyses in relation to body mass and composition: Research from whole-body CT scans of adult humans. *Am. J. Phys. Anthropol.* **2018**, *167*, 813–826. [CrossRef]
65. Ruff, C.B. New approaches to structural evolution of limb bones in primates. *Folia Primatol.* **1989**, *53*, 142–159. [CrossRef]
66. Ruff, C.B.; Hayes, W.C. Cross-sectional geometry of Pecos Pueblo femora and tibiae—A biomechanical investigation: I. Method and general patterns of variation. *Am. J. Phys. Anthropol.* **1983**, *60*, 359–381. [CrossRef]
67. Sládek, V.; Berner, M.; Sailer, R. Mobility in central European late Eneolithic and early bronze age: Femoral cross-sectional geometry. *Am. J. Phys. Anthropol.* **2006**, *130*, 320–332. [CrossRef]
68. Lieberman, D.E.; Polk, J.D.; Demes, B. Predicting long bone loading from cross-sectional geometry. *Am. J. Phys. Anthropol.* **2004**, *123*, 156–171. [CrossRef]
69. Koso, R.E.; Terhoeve, C.; Steen, R.G.; Zura, R. Healing, nonunion, and re-operation after internal fixation of diaphyseal and distal femoral fractures: A systematic review and meta-analysis. *Int. Orthop.* **2018**, *42*, 2675–2683. [CrossRef]

Disclaimer/Publisher's Note: The statements, opinions and data contained in all publications are solely those of the individual author(s) and contributor(s) and not of MDPI and/or the editor(s). MDPI and/or the editor(s) disclaim responsibility for any injury to people or property resulting from any ideas, methods, instructions or products referred to in the content.

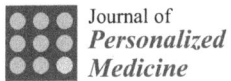

Communication

Results of Treating Mild to Moderate Knee Osteoarthritis with Autologous Conditioned Adipose Tissue and Leukocyte-Poor Platelet-Rich Plasma

Vilim Molnar [1,2], Eduard Pavelić [1], Željko Jeleč [1,3], Petar Brlek [1], Vid Matišić [1], Igor Borić [1,4,5], Damir Hudetz [1,2,6], Eduard Rod [1], Dinko Vidović [1,7,8], Neven Starčević [1], Martin Čemerin [9], David C. Karli [10] and Dragan Primorac [1,2,4,11,12,13,14,15,16,*]

1. St. Catherine Specialty Hospital, 10000 Zagreb, Croatia
2. Faculty of Medicine, Josip Juraj Strossmayer University of Osijek, 31000 Osijek, Croatia
3. Department of Nursing, University North, 42000 Varaždin, Croatia
4. School of Medicine, University of Split, 21000 Split, Croatia
5. Department of Health Studies, University of Split, 21000 Split, Croatia
6. Department for Traumatology and Orthopaedics, University Hospital Dubrava, 10000 Zagreb, Croatia
7. Clinic for Traumatology, University Hospital "Sisters of Mercy", 10000 Zagreb, Croatia
8. School of Dental Medicine, University of Zagreb, 10000 Zagreb, Croatia
9. School of Medicine, University of Zagreb, 10000 Zagreb, Croatia
10. The Steadman Clinic, Vail, CO 81657, USA
11. School of Medicine, Faculty of Dental Medicine and Health, Josip Juraj Strossmayer University Osijek, 31000 Osijek, Croatia
12. Medical School, University of Rijeka, 51000 Rijeka, Croatia
13. Medical School, University of Mostar, 88000 Mostar, Bosnia and Herzegovina
14. Eberly College of Science, Penn State University, 517 Thomas St., State College, PA 16803, USA
15. The Henry C Lee College of Criminal Justice & Forensic Sciences, University of New Haven, West Haven, CT 06516, USA
16. Medical School REGIOMED, 96450 Coburg, Germany
* Correspondence: draganprimorac2@gmail.com

Abstract: Knee osteoarthritis (KOA) is one of the most common musculoskeletal disorders. Much progress has been made in regenerative medicine for the symptomatic treatment of KOA, including products containing stromal vascular fraction (SVF) and platelet-rich plasma (PRP). The aim of this study was to evaluate clinical and radiological findings after the application of autologous conditioned adipose tissue (ACA) and leukocyte-poor PRP (LP-PRP) in patients with mild to moderate KOA. A total of 16 patients (eight male and eight female) with changes related to KOA on the magnetic resonance imaging (MRI), but without severe osteophytosis, full-thickness cartilage loss, or subchondral bone involvement were included in this study. Patients received an intraarticular, ultrasound-guided injection of ACA and LP-PRP. Clinical scores, including a visual analog scale for pain (VAS), Knee Injury and Osteoarthritis Outcome Score (KOOS), and Western Ontario and McMaster Universities Osteoarthritis Index (WOMAC) were evaluated at baseline and at the three and six month follow-ups showing a statistically significant improvements at three and six months post-intervention. Furthermore, the delayed gadolinium-enhanced MRI of the cartilage (dGEMRIC) indices were evaluated at baseline and at the three and six month follow-ups showing no significant changes after treatment with ACA and LP-PRP, which were actually equal to the dGEMRIC indices measured in the control group (hyaluronic acid applied in contralateral knees without osteoarthritis). ACA with LP-PRP presents a viable minimally invasive therapeutic option for the clinical improvement of mild to moderate KOA. However, MFAT produced by different systems is likely to differ in cellular content, which can directly affect the paracrine effect (cytokine secretion) of mesenchymal stem cells and consequently the regeneration process.

Keywords: knee osteoarthritis; mesenchymal stem cells; stromal vascular fraction; adipose tissue; platelet-rich plasma

Citation: Molnar, V.; Pavelić, E.; Jeleč, Ž.; Brlek, P.; Matišić, V.; Borić, I.; Hudetz, D.; Rod, E.; Vidović, D.; Starčević, N.; et al. Results of Treating Mild to Moderate Knee Osteoarthritis with Autologous Conditioned Adipose Tissue and Leukocyte-Poor Platelet-Rich Plasma. *J. Pers. Med.* **2023**, *13*, 47. https://doi.org/10.3390/jpm13010047

Academic Editors: Nan Jiang and Weikuan Gu

Received: 26 October 2022
Revised: 5 December 2022
Accepted: 21 December 2022
Published: 26 December 2022

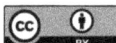

Copyright: © 2022 by the authors. Licensee MDPI, Basel, Switzerland. This article is an open access article distributed under the terms and conditions of the Creative Commons Attribution (CC BY) license (https://creativecommons.org/licenses/by/4.0/).

1. Introduction

Osteoarthritis (OA) is one of the most common musculoskeletal pathologies with over 654 million patients worldwide, while this number is expected to rise due to an aging and a progressively obese world population [1]. It affects 21.7% of women and 11.9% of men over 40 years of age. The most predominantly affected joint in OA is the knee [2]. The high prevalence of this disease in older population groups, and the immense costs associated with this disease create a precarious situation for healthcare systems to find more affordable alternatives [3,4]. Due to the inefficiencies of the current nonoperative treatment of OA, there is a financial burden on both the patient and the healthcare system [4,5].

In recent years orthobiologic therapies offered great potential in the treatment of OA [6]. Options, such as the application of stromal vascular fraction (SVF) and microfragmented adipose tissue (MFAT) have shown encouraging results in the treatment of patients with knee osteoarthritis (KOA), including clinical and radiological improvements [7–10]. SVF is obtained through either mechanical or enzymatic degradation of lipoaspirate. Enzymatically, SVF can be obtained with the use of collagenase and centrifugation. Still the subject of discussion, mechanical isolation of SVF can be performed through a combination of centrifugation and intersyringe processing. Both methods have proven similar chondrogenic potentials in vivo [11]. If obtained correctly, SVF has shown excellent clinical results with a significant reduction in pain scores [12–15].

The alternative biological method that has been widely used in the past decade is the application of platelet-rich plasma (PRP). To be considered PRP, the platelet concentration must be 1,000,000 platelets/µL in a 5 mL volume of plasma [16]. However, there is significant heterogeneity in preparation systems of PRP, such as leukocyte-rich, leukocyte-poor PRP (LP-PRP), and others [17–19]. The plethora of growth factors present in PRP makes it an excellent therapeutic tool in the treatment of KOA [17,20–22]. Although PRP has shown great clinical results for patients with mild to moderate KOA, the current school of thought is to combine the two therapeutic methods to create a synergistic effect.

The aim of this study was to evaluate the effects of combination therapy with autologous conditioned adipose tissue containing SVF (ACA-SVF) and adjunct LP-PRP for mild to moderate KOA.

2. Materials and Methods

2.1. Study Design

This prospective, non-randomized, interventional, single-center, and open-label clinical study involved patients with primarily mild to moderate KOA who received a combination of ACA and LP-PRP. Mild to moderate KOA is defined as the presence of osteoarthritic knee changes but without diffuse full-thickness cartilage loss with underlying subchondral bone reactive changes in any joint surfaces (grade IV defects according to the International Cartilage Research Society (ICRS) based on the modified Outerbridge system). Clinical results were noted by filling out clinical questionnaires prior to intervention and 3 and 6 months after the intervention. All patients signed informed consent before being included in the study. The study was conducted in St. Catherine Specialty Hospital, Zabok, Croatia. We confirm that all methods were performed following the relevant guidelines and regulations. The study was approved by the St. Catherine's Ethical Committee, authorization No: 21/3-1.

2.2. Participants

A total of 16 patients (8 male and 8 female) with KOA were included in this study. All the study participants were clinically examined by an orthopedic surgeon, and a magnetic resonance imaging (MRI) of the affected knee was performed along with standard knee X-rays. Unaffected knees, without KOA (contralateral knees of the same patients) were treated with hyaluronic acid (HA) (Hyalubrix® 60, Fidia Farmaceutici S.P.A., Abano Terme, Italy) to compare the dGEMRIC indices with knees with KOA treated with ACA and LP-PRP.

Patient inclusion and exclusion criteria are described in Table 1.

Table 1. Patient inclusion and exclusion criteria.

Patient inclusion criteria	1. 2.	patients with KOA patients older than 18 years and younger than 75 years
Patient exclusion criteria	• • • • • • • •	patients with malignant disease patients with systemic inflammatory diseases (e.g., rheumatoid arthritis) patients with diffuse grade IV chondromalacia according to the ICRS classification patients with an unstable knee on clinical exam or with visible anterior cruciate ligament tear on MRI patients with acute meniscal lesions or injuries of other knee structures as the main cause of pain and other symptoms patients with a history of knee surgery patients with mental illness (patients in whom cooperation cannot be expected during the study) patients who are found to be unable to respond to follow-up examinations

2.3. Clinical Questionnaires

All patients were screened by an orthopedic examination following which they answered the orthopedic questionnaires related to KOA: the KOOS (Knee Injury and Osteoarthritis Outcome Score), the WOMAC (Western Ontario and McMaster Universities Osteoarthritis Index), and the pain level was assessed using a visual analog scale (VAS). For patients that were included in this study, clinical questionnaires were assessed at baseline and 3 and 6 months after the intervention. In the follow-up period, the patients were instructed to maintain normal daily activities.

2.4. Delayed Gadolinium-Enhanced Magnetic Resonance Imaging of Cartilage (dGEMRIC) Protocol

MR imaging was performed on a 1.5 T magnet (Avanto; Siemens, Erlangen, Germany) using a dedicated knee coil (Siemens, Erlangen, Germany). The severity of early OA in this study cohort was determined, according to the MRI, by an experienced musculoskeletal radiologist using the scoring system introduced by the International Cartilage Research Society (ICRS) based on the modified Outerbridge system.

After the completion of the clinical examination and the questionnaires, the patients were given intravenous contrast (gadolinium) to perform dGEMRIC.

Each subject received gadolinium diethylene triamine penta-acetic acid (Dotarem; Guerbet, Roissy CgG Cedex, Villepinte, France), 0.2 mmol/kg, administered with an injection time of less than 5 min through an IV infusion catheter placed in the antecubital vein with the patient in the supine position. The administered MRI contrast agent was the same for all patients because the MRI contrast agent was always applied under the same conditions: contrast agent temperature, magnetic field strength, and contrast agent concentration. The subjects waited 5 min after injection, then exercised by walking up and down the stairs and continued to walk on a flat surface for approximately 10 min to stimulate delivery of the contrast agent to the joint. Post-contrast imaging of the cartilage was performed 60 min after contrast administration. The dGEMRIC index was obtained by an experienced musculoskeletal radiologist using syngoMaplt software (Siemens, Erlangen, Germany). Seven different articular facets were analyzed, and the dGEMRIC index was calculated: the medial and lateral femoral condyle, femoral trochlea, medial and lateral tibial condyle, and both patellar facets, before the intra-articular application of stem cells and in any subsequent MRI examination at 3, and 6 months after the intra-articular application of ACA-SVF and LP-PRP. Regions of interest (ROIs), in which an average dGEMRIC index was calculated, were manually drawn to consistently cover the same weight-bearing part of each articular cartilage facet. Articular facets on which the dGEMRIC index was not measured were labeled as "-".

2.5. Lipoaspiration and ACA Production

The patients were referred to the day surgery unit with an average admission of three hours. The surgical part of the procedure was performed in an operating theater. The patients were placed in a supine position; the abdominal skin was treated with antiseptic lotion Dermoguard® (Antiseptica, Pulheim, Germany), rinsed with *Aqua pro injectione* solution (HZTM, Zagreb, Croatia), dried out, and disinfected with Skin-Des® solution (Antiseptica, Pulheim, Germany). Injection of 2% lidocaine was administered to the incision site, after which a 2–3 mm incision was made. The minimally invasive surgical procedure included an infiltration step, in which a total of 250 mL of the saline solution was prepared with a 40 mL of a 2% lidocaine solution (Lidokain®, Belupo, Koprivnica, Croatia) and 1 mL epinephrine hydrochloride (1 mg/mL) (Suprarenin®, Sanofi-Aventis, Berlin, Germany) was injected into the abdominal subcutaneous adipose tissue. In the aspiration step, a standard lipoaspiration technique was performed, and the harvested fat was collected by a Carraway Harvester (2.1 mm × 15 cm) connected to a VacLock syringe (Arthrex, Munich, Germany) that was inserted through a small stab incision where up to 60 mL of adipose tissue was collected into the syringe by the vacuum created by the system. Steristrips (3M) were taped, and compression bandages were applied over the incisions to prevent hematoma formation.

The obtained lipoaspirate was divided into several (up to 4) separate syringes (Arthrex ACP® Double-Syringe System (Arthrex, Munich, Germany)) and centrifuged for 4 min at 2500 rpm. Upon completion of centrifugation, 3 layers within the syringe were distinguished. The lowest layer, the aqueous fraction, was poured out, while the highest layer, the layer of broken adipocyte oil, was removed using the Arthrex ACP® Double-Syringe System. The middle layer, a layer of autologous conditioned adipose tissue (ACA), was mixed with the same layers of the other syringes through a 1.4 mm wide transfer device at least 30 times to obtain a homogenized adipose tissue product (ACA Microfat). ACA Microfat was centrifuged again for 4 min at 2500 rpm. Again, the oil, which was in the upper layer, was separated and discarded, and the aqueous fraction poured out. The middle layer, consisting of ACA-SVF containing adipose-derived mesenchymal stem cells, was used as the final product for application to the patient's knee joint. All the patients received 2 mL of ACA-SVF in combination with LP-PRP.

2.6. LP-PRP Protocol

A 90 mL sample of venous blood was taken from the patient to prepare LP-PRP using the Arthrex Angel System™. The settings were adjusted to increase the number of platelets to 5.57-fold while keeping the leukocyte and neutrophil levels at 0.78 and 0.53 in relation to normal venous blood. The final LP-PRP volume was set to 5 mL. In patients where less than 5 mL of LP-PRP was obtained, platelet-poor plasma (PPP) was added to the mixture so that the final volume was equal to 5 mL.

2.7. Application of ACA + LP-PRP

Finally, the ACA (2 mL) was mixed with LP-PRP (5 mL) to form the final product. After disinfection of the puncture site, a 21-gauge needle was inserted into the synovial space of the knee joint guided by ultrasound. Synovial fluid was drawn from the knee, and a combination of ACA and LP-PRP was injected through the same needle used to aspirate the synovial fluid. Upon completion of the procedure, patients spent approximately 2 h in the hospital and were discharged home afterward.

2.8. Follow-Up Appointments

All patients arrived for a follow-up examination 3 and 6 months after the initial treatment. During these intervals, patients underwent magnetic resonance imaging (dGEMRIC) of the knee to determine the morphological and molecular state of the cartilage and its response to the combined ACA and LP-PRP therapy. Afterward, the patients answered the orthopedic questionnaires (VAS, KOOS, and WOMAC) to compare the clinical findings with the results before the initial treatment, thus assessing the clinical response to the ACA and LP-PRP therapy.

2.9. Statistical Analysis

A statistical analysis of the obtained data was performed in the software package IBM SPSS Statistics 23.0 (SPSS, Chicago, IL, USA). Graphs were created in GraphPad Prism version 9.4.1. for Windows (GraphPad Software, San Diego, CA, USA). Descriptive statistical methods were used to describe the frequency of the investigated variables. The normality of the distribution of the variables was tested by the Kolmogorov–Smirnov test. We used Friedman's test to compare three or more paired groups and the Wilcoxon matched pairs test to determine the differences between two paired groups (repeated measurements within the same group of subjects).

3. Results

3.1. Visual Analog Scale (VAS)

Patients were followed-up at three and six months for a score assessment during rest and movement. The results demonstrated no statistical difference in VAS scores between the two genders. However, there was a statistically significant VAS improvement in response to therapy at three and six months at both rest and during movement (Figure 1, Table 2). The mean scores for VAS in rest decreased from 3.00 to 1.00 at three months and then finally to 0.50 at six months. The mean scores for VAS in movement decreased from 6.00 to 2.00 at three and six months after the intervention.

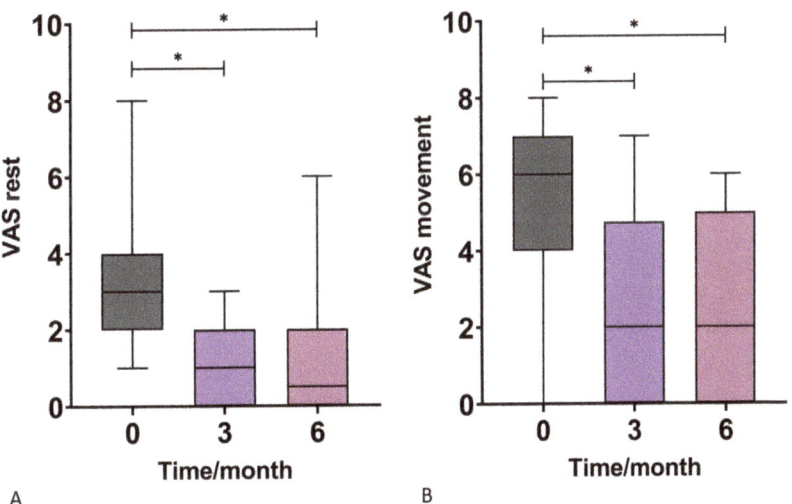

Figure 1. Box-plots show the distribution of visual analog scale (VAS) scores for pain in rest (**A**) and movement (**B**) at baseline and at 3 and 6 months after the application of autologous conditioned adipose tissue and leukocyte-poor platelet-rich plasma. Statistically significant VAS improvement in response to therapy was observed at 3 and 6 months at both rest and during movement. *—$p < 0.05$ (Wilcoxon test).

Table 2. Median values of VAS, KOOS, and WOMAC scores. M—median; IQR—interquartile range; SD—standard deviation; T0—baseline score; T3—score after 3 months; T6—score after 6 months; VAS—Visual analog scale; KOOS—Knee Injury and Osteoarthritis Outcome Score; WOMAC—Western Ontario and McMaster Universities Osteoarthritis Index.

		T0	T3	T6	p Value (Kruskal-Wallis Test)
VAS-Rest	M	3.00	1.00	0.50	<0.001
	IQR	2.00	2.00	2.00	
	SD	±1.797	±1.063	±1.628	
VAS-Active	M	6.00	2.00	2.00	0.002
	IQR	3.00	4.75	5.00	
	SD	±2.066	±2.613	±2.277	
KOOS Symptoms	M	76.79	94.64	100.00	0.001
	IQR	21.43	21.43	16.96	
	SD	±16.24	±10.93	±9.873	
KOOS Pain	M	65.28	81.94	90.28	0.017
	IQR	40.28	25.00	30.56	
	SD	±21.42	±15.00	±17.22	
KOOS Activities of Daily Living	M	75.00	89.71	96.32	0.014
	IQR	34.93	23.16	24.26	
	SD	±20.00	±14.91	±15.37	
KOOS Sport and Recreation Function	M	27.50	55.00	70.00	0.006
	IQR	56.25	58.75	63.75	
	SD	±28.72	±29.71	±29.42	
KOOS Quality of Life	M	37.50	50.00	53.13	0.064
	IQR	29.69	54.69	43.75	
	SD	±26.81	±29.75	±27.28	
WOMAC Pain	M	5.00	1.50	1.00	0.009
	IQR	8.00	6.75	4.50	
	SD	±4.423	±3.637	±3.856	
WOMAC Stiffness	M	2.00	0.00	0.00	0.014
	IQR	3.00	2.75	1.50	
	SD	±2.160	±1.455	±1.559	
WOMAC Function	M	18.50	5.00	2.50	0.006
	IQR	19.00	14.50	12.75	
	SD	±10.92	±9.793	±9.858	
Total WOMAC	M	27.50	7.50	4.00	0.005
	IQR	24.00	20.50	23.25	
	SD	±15.75	±13.87	±14.08	

Table 2. Cont.

		T0	T3	T6	p Value (Kruskal-Wallis Test)
		T0	T3	T6	p value (Friedman test)
VAS-Rest	M	3	1	0.5	<0.0001
	IQR	2	2	2	
	SD	±1.797	±1.063	±1.628	
VAS-Active	M	6	2	2	<0.0001
	IQR	3	4.75	5	
	SD	±2.066	±2.613	±2.277	
KOOS Symptoms	M	76.79	94.64	100	<0.0001
	IQR	21.43	21.43	16.96	
	SD	±16.24	±10.93	±9.873	
KOOS Pain	M	65.28	81.94	90.28	<0.0001
	IQR	40.28	25	30.56	
	SD	±21.42	±15.00	±17.22	
KOOS Activities of Daily Living	M	75	89.71	96.32	0.0001
	IQR	34.93	23.16	24.26	
	SD	±20.00	±14.91	±15.37	
KOOS Sport and Recreation Function	M	27.5	55	70	<0.0001
	IQR	56.25	58.75	63.75	
	SD	±28.72	±29.71	±29.42	
KOOS Quality of Life	M	37.5	50	53.13	0.0004
	IQR	29.69	54.69	43.75	
	SD	±26.81	±29.75	±27.28	
WOMAC Pain	M	5	1.5	1	<0.0001
	IQR	8	6.75	4.5	
	SD	±4.423	±3.637	±3.856	
WOMAC Stiffness	M	2	0	0	<0.0001
	IQR	3	2.75	1.5	
	SD	±2.160	±1.455	±1.559	
WOMAC Function	M	18.5	5	2.5	0.0003
	IQR	19	14.5	12.75	
	SD	±10.92	±9.793	±9.858	
Total WOMAC	M	27.5	7.5	4	0.0002
	IQR	24	20.5	23.25	
	SD	±15.75	±13.87	±14.08	

3.2. Knee Injury and Osteoarthritis Outcome Score (KOOS)

There were statistically significant increases in the KOOS symptoms subscores across all time points (three and six months) when compared to the baseline score before intervention. The median value steeply increased from the baseline of 76.79 to 94.64 at three months and finally reached 100.00 at the end of the six month follow-up (Figure 2A, Table 2). Furthermore, a statistically significant increase was observed in the KOOS pain scores at three and six months when compared to the baseline score before intervention. A steady increase from the median baseline value of 65.28 to 81.94 at three months and then 90.28 was noted (Figure 2B, Table 2). A statistically significant increases in the KOOS Activities of Daily Living subscore were observed after the therapeutic intervention when compared to the baseline scores. The mean scores increased from 75.00 to 89.71 at three months and then finally to 96.32 at six months (Figure 2C, Table 2). The KOOS Sport and Recreation Function subscore was also found to be statistically significant by the increase in values when compared to the baseline scores (Figure 2D, Table 2). Median values rose from 27.50 to 55.00 at the three months follow-up and at six months it increased further to 70.00. Increases in KOOS Quality of Life subscores values were found (Figure 2E, Table 2). A statistically significant improvement in the KOOS Quality of life score was observed by a rise in median values from the baseline 37.50 to 50.00 at three months and 53.13 at the six months follow-up.

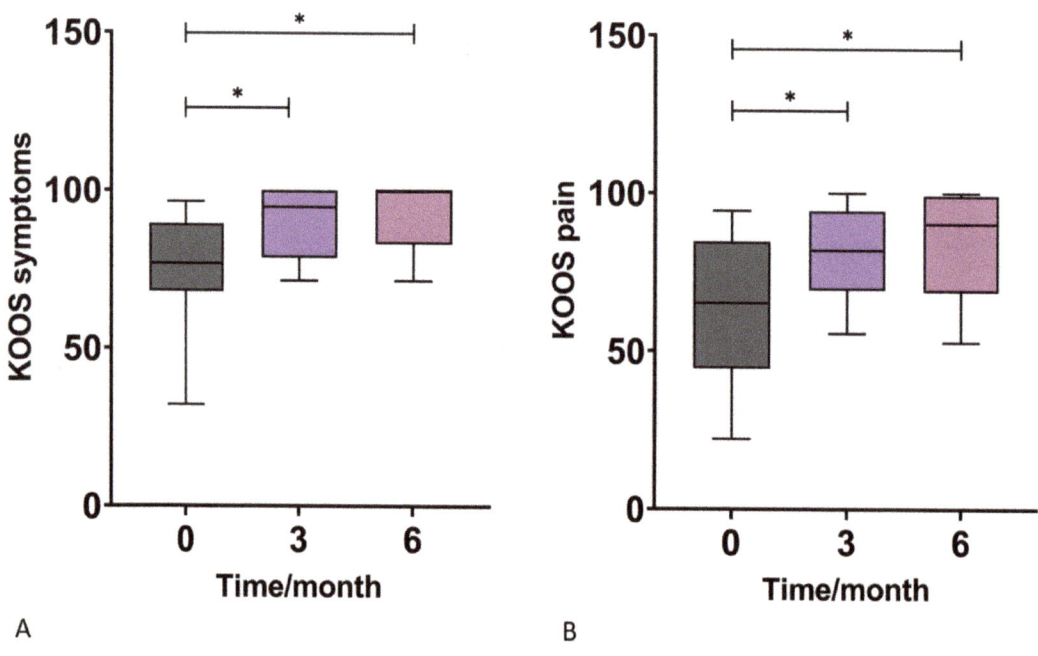

Figure 2. *Cont.*

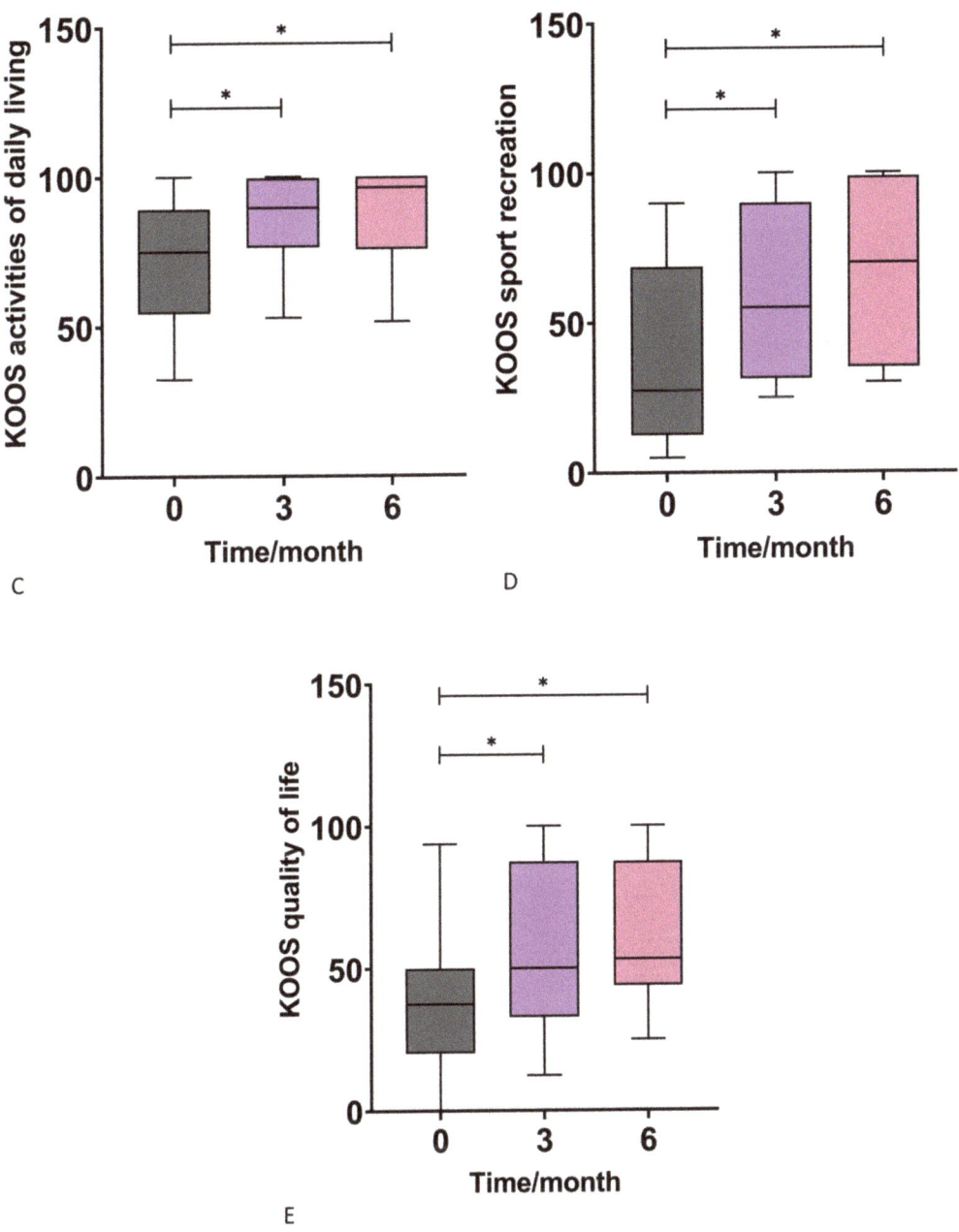

Figure 2. Box-plots show the distribution of Knee Injury and Osteoarthritis Outcome Scores (KOOS) subscores for symptoms (**A**), pain (**B**), activities of daily living (**C**), sport and recreation function (**D**), and quality of life (**E**) at baseline and at 3 and 6 months after application of autologous conditioned adipose tissue and leukocyte-poor platelet-rich plasma. There was a significant improvement in all subscores at 3 and 6 months after the therapeutic intervention when compared to the baseline. *—$p < 0.05$ (Wilcoxon test).

3.3. Western Ontario and McMaster Universities Osteoarthritis Index (WOMAC)

There was a statistically significant decrease in the WOMAC pain subscores across all time points (three and six months) when compared to the baseline score before intervention. The median value steeply decreased from the baseline of 5.00 to 1.50 at three months and reached 1.00 at the end of the 6-month follow-up (Figure 3A, Table 2). Furthermore, a statistically significant decrease was observed in the WOMAC Stiffness scores at three and six months when compared to the baseline score. A decrease from the median baseline value of 2.00 to 0.00 at three and six months was noted (Figure 3B, Table 2). A statistically significant decrease in the WOMAC function subscore was observed after the therapeutic intervention when compared to the baseline scores. The mean scores decreased from 18.50 to 5.00 at three months and then to 2.50 at six months (Figure 3C, Table 2). Finally, the total WOMAC score significantly decreased from the median baseline value of 27.50 to 7.50 three months after the intervention and to 4.00 at the six month follow-up (Figure 3D, Table 2).

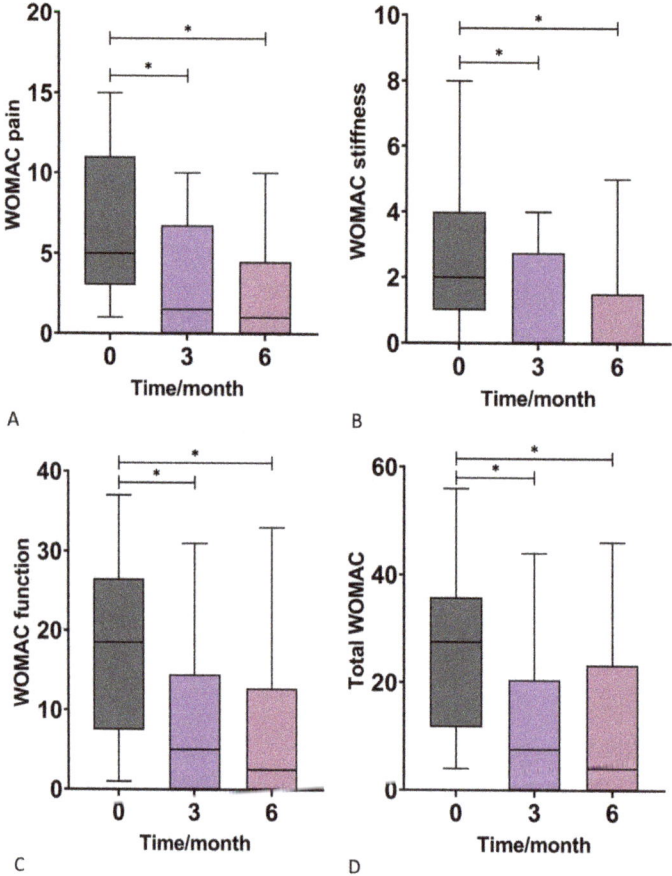

Figure 3. Box-plots show the distribution of Western Ontario and McMaster Universities Osteoarthritis Index (WOMAC) subscores for pain (**A**), stiffness (**B**), function (**C**), and the total score (**D**) at baseline and at 3 and 6 months after application of autologous conditioned adipose tissue and leukocyte-poor platelet-rich plasma. There was a significant improvement in all subscores 3 and 6 months after the therapeutic intervention compared to the baseline. *—$p < 0.05$ (Wilcoxon test).

3.4. dGEMRIC

The magnetic resonance imaging using the dGEMRIC index showed no significant improvement in the glycosaminoglycan (GAG) composition of the cartilage in the knees treated with ACA-SVF and LP-PRP at 3- and 6-month follow-ups when compared to the baseline values for each of the analyzed compartments, including medial and lateral femur, medial and lateral tibia, trochlea, and medial and lateral patella (Figure 4).

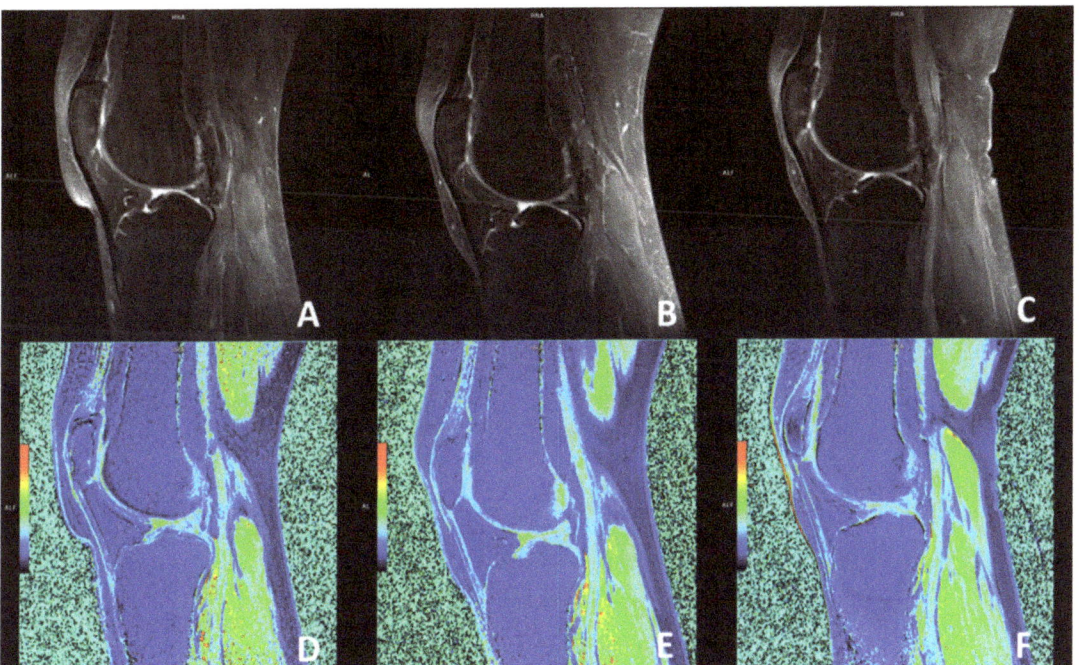

Figure 4. Sagittal MRI magnetic resonance imaging (MRI) slices through the center of the knee accessing the patellofemoral joint osteoarthritic changes using fat-suppressed proton-density-weighted turbo spin-echo method at baseline (**A**), 3 months (**B**), and 6 months (**C**) follow-ups with corresponding delayed gadolinium-enhanced MRI of the cartilage (dGEMRIC) images (**D**–**F**). No changes were seen when dGEMRIC indices were calculated.

4. Discussion

The results of the presented study indicate that patients experienced statistically significant clinical improvements, as seen in the reduction in the VAS and WOMAC scores and the increase in KOOS from the baseline values to the follow-up periods of three and six months. These changes were observed in the total test scores and in the test subcategories. This is in line with previous studies [23–27]. It was shown earlier that SVF and PRP can influence paracrine activity through the various factors secreted, which include: PDGF, TGF, VEGF, EGF, FGF, CTGF, IGF-1, HGF, KGF, Ang-1, PF4, SDF-1, and TNF [17,28–30]. It is the presence of these factors that are responsible for the anti-inflammatory effects and are the likely contributors to the improved scores at three and six months [17,28–30]. According to Baria et al. a patient's degree of activity before the treatment could influence the clinical outcomes because it could influence the PRP content [31]. In our research, the physical activity of patients was not reported before the study. Previous research with MFAT has shown a statistical improvement in the dGEMRIC values indirectly showing the glycosaminoglycan (GAG) concentration in the hyaline cartilage [9,10]. However, this was not observed in the present study. A possible hypothesis explaining this observation might lay in the quantitative presence of MSCs in MFAT when compared to that of ACA.

While the work by Zenić et al. proved that the same population of cells (after treating the samples with 1% collagenase type I) is present in identical ratios in both MFAT and ACA, the results in this study might be explained by the ACA method used in this study as an inefficient methodology in obtaining a significant amount of SVF or by the insufficient cell quantity. [32]. In addition, the total cellular count obtained by the ACA method used in this study (2 mL) may be less in comparison with the larger volume samples of MFAT from other systems. Available SVF, as well as a larger quantity of cells could directly influence cartilage regeneration However, there is no consensus on the dosage of MSCs [33]. Low and high dosages have both been proven to have a beneficial effect [34]. Gupta et al. showed that the optimal dose of BM-MSCs might be around 25×10^6 cells, while higher doses were associated with higher adverse events [35]. Other studies have found that doses between 2×10^6 and 60×10^6 of MSCs, when applied at a greater frequency, were potentially within a therapeutic range [36]. Eventually, the paracrine effect of MSCs derived from adipose tissue plays a critical role in cartilage regeneration. Additionally, there is no doubt that the MFAT produced by different systems is likely to differ in cellular content, which can directly affect the paracrine effect (cytokine secretion) of mesenchymal stem cells.

Furthermore, Chalal et al. found that higher doses of 50×10^6 BM-MSCs resulted in a lessening of synovitis and an improvement in the WOMAC scores [37]. Another possible hypothesis is that the perivascular milieu is less disrupted in MFAT than in ACA-SVF. As evidenced, pericytes are an in vivo origin of MSCs and play a role in the chondrogenic potentials of MSCs [38,39]. Therefore, a less disrupted milieu due to minimal manipulation, or centrifugation, might result in a better function of this important cell group and thus result in better a chondrogenic potential in vivo [40,41]. However, collagenase-derived SVF preparations were shown to have a greater chondrogenic potential in vitro than their mechanically derived counterparts [11,42]. Accordingly, a direct comparison of different SVF results might lead to false conclusions as the method of extraction in the majority of research is not clearly identified. However, similar results to MFAT were seen when comparing studies using enzymatically prepared SVF [12–15]. As such, the clinical effects of ACA-SVF with LP-PRP therapy could be the result of the anti-inflammatory effects from the cells and growth factors present [42,43]. Further building on these findings, several studies have concluded that a more standardized approach should be conducted in terms of which PRP formulation should be used [43], intending to answer questions posed by currently available guidelines and with the goal of an eventual inclusion in the guidelines [17,33].

The limitations of this study include a small patient size (the reason for which the study did not consider age and BMI in the interpretation of results). A further limitation is the addition to the LP-PRP with PPP to fulfill the volume deficit in the final end product and an undetermined amount of MSCs that were delivered intraarticularly. The latter is a constant limiting factor in all the studies in this field, which should be defined in further work.

5. Conclusions

A combination therapy of ACA and LP-PRP provides excellent clinical and statistically significant improvements in symptoms in patients with mild to moderate KOA. Overall, the growing body of evidence supports SVF with PRP as a minimally invasive approach in the management of KOA. However, the cellular composition of MFAT plays a critical role in cartilage regeneration. Mesenchymal stem cells from adipose tissue provide an excellent safety profile and favorable outcomes for patients based on observed pain and joint function. However, there needs to be a more structured experimental approach, along with standardization of the terminology concerning the application of all forms of MSCs and the objectification of outcomes. Furthermore, a more structured selection of patients regarding KOA staging is necessary before making a final conclusion.

Author Contributions: Conceptualization, V.M. (Vilim Molnar) and D.P.; methodology, V.M. (Vilim Molnar), Ž.J., V.M. (Vid Matišić), I.B., D.H., E.R., D.V., N.S. and M.Č.; investigation, V.M. (Vilim Molnar), V.M. (Vid Matišić) and M.Č.; writing—original draft preparation, (Vilim Molnar), E.P., P.B., V.M. (Vid Matišić) and M.Č.; writing—review and editing, Ž.J., D.H., E.R., D.V., D.C.K. and D.P.; visualization, P.B.; supervision, D.P. All authors have read and agreed to the published version of the manuscript.

Funding: This research received no external funding.

Institutional Review Board Statement: The study was conducted in accordance with the Declaration of Helsinki, and approved by the Ethics Committee of St. Catherine Specialty Hospital (protocol code 21/3-1, 9 March 2021).

Informed Consent Statement: Informed consent was obtained from all subjects involved in the study. Written informed consent has been obtained from the patients to publish this paper.

Data Availability Statement: The data presented in this study are available on request from the corresponding author.

Acknowledgments: We thank the International Society for Applied Biological Sciences (ISABS) for their continuing support for our research on mesenchymal stem cells.

Conflicts of Interest: The authors declare no conflict of interest.

References

1. Cui, A.; Li, H.; Wang, D.; Zhong, J.; Chen, Y.; Lu, H. EClinicalMedicine Global, regional prevalence, incidence and risk factors of knee osteoarthritis in population-based studies. *EClinicalMedicine* **2020**, *29*, 100587. [CrossRef] [PubMed]
2. Hunter, D.J.; Bierma-Zeinstra, S. Osteoarthritis. *Lancet* **2019**, *393*, 1745–1759. [CrossRef] [PubMed]
3. Uhlig, T.; Slatkowsky-Christensen, B.; Moe, R.H.; Kvien, T.K. The burden of osteoarthritis: The societal and the patient perspective. *Therapy* **2010**, *7*, 605–619. [CrossRef]
4. Losina, E.; Paltiel, A.D.; Weinstein, A.M.; Yelin, E.; Hunter, D.J.; Chen, S.P.; Klara, K.; Suter, L.G.; Solomon, D.H.; Burbine, S.A.; et al. Lifetime medical costs of knee osteoarthritis management in the United States: Impact of extending indications for total knee arthroplasty. *Arthritis Care Res.* **2015**, *67*, 203–215. [CrossRef]
5. Lanes, S.F.; Lanza, L.L.; Radensky, P.W.; Yood, R.A.; Meenan, R.F.; Walker, A.M.; Dreyer, N.A. Resource utilization and cost of care for rheumatoid arthritis and osteoarthritis in a managed care setting: The importance of drug and surgery costs. *Arthritis Rheum.* **1997**, *40*, 1475–1481. [CrossRef]
6. Primorac, D.; Molnar, V.; Rod, E.; Jeleč, Ž.; Čukelj, F.; Matišić, V.; Vrdoljak, T.; Hudetz, D.; Hajsok, H.; Borić, I. Knee Osteoarthritis: A Review of Pathogenesis and State-Of-The-Art Non-Operative Therapeutic Considerations. *Genes* **2020**, *11*, 854. [CrossRef]
7. Hudetz, D.; Borić, I.; Rod, E.; Jeleč, Ž.; Kunovac, B.; Polašek, O.; Vrdoljak, T.; Plečko, M.; Skelin, A.; Polančec, D.; et al. Early results of intra-articular micro-fragmented lipoaspirate treatment in patients with late stages knee osteoarthritis: A prospective study. *Croat. Med. J.* **2019**, *60*, 227–236. [CrossRef]
8. Hudetz, D.; Jeleč, Ž.; Rod, E.; Borić, I.; Plečko, M.; Primorac, D. The Future of Cartilage Repair. *Pers. Med. Healthc. Syst.* **2019**, *5*, 375–411. [CrossRef]
9. Hudetz, D.; Borić, I.; Rod, E.; Jeleč, Ž.; Radić, A.; Vrdoljak, T.; Skelin, A.; Lauc, G.; Trbojević-Akmačić, I.; Plečko, M.; et al. The effect of intra-articular injection of autologous microfragmented fat tissue on proteoglycan synthesis in patients with knee osteoarthritis. *Genes* **2017**, *8*, 270. [CrossRef] [PubMed]
10. Borić, I.; Hudetz, D.; Rod, E.; Jeleč, Ž.; Vrdoljak, T.; Skelin, A.; Polašek, O.; Plečko, M.; Trbojević-Akmačić, I.; Lauc, G.; et al. A 24-month follow-up study of the effect of intra-articular injection of autologous microfragmented fat tissue on proteoglycan synthesis in patients with knee osteoarthritis. *Genes* **2019**, *10*, 1051. [CrossRef]
11. Chaput, B.; Bertheuil, N.; Escubes, M.; Grolleau, J.L.; Garrido, I.; Laloze, J.; Espagnolle, N.; Casteilla, L.; Sensebé, L.; Varin, A. Mechanically Isolated Stromal Vascular Fraction Provides a Valid and Useful Collagenase-Free Alternative Technique: A Comparative Study. *Plast. Reconstr. Surg.* **2016**, *138*, 807–819. [CrossRef] [PubMed]
12. Kim, Y.S.; Choi, Y.J.; Suh, D.S.; Heo, D.B.; Kim, Y.I.; Ryu, J.S.; Koh, Y.G. Mesenchymal stem cell implantation in osteoarthritic knees: Is fibrin glue effective as a scaffold? *Am. J. Sport. Med.* **2015**, *43*, 176–185. [CrossRef] [PubMed]
13. Tsubosaka, M.; Matsumoto, T.; Sobajima, S.; Matsushita, T.; Iwaguro, H.; Kuroda, R. The influence of adipose-derived stromal vascular fraction cells on the treatment of knee osteoarthritis. *BMC Musculoskelet. Disord.* **2020**, *21*, 207. [CrossRef] [PubMed]
14. Hong, Z.; Chen, J.; Zhang, S.; Zhao, C.; Bi, M.; Chen, X.; Bi, Q. Intra-articular injection of autologous adipose-derived stromal vascular fractions for knee osteoarthritis: A double-blind randomized self-controlled trial. *Int. Orthop.* **2019**, *43*, 1123–1134. [CrossRef] [PubMed]
15. Fodor, P.B.; Paulseth, S.G. Adipose Derived Stromal Cell (ADSC) Injections for Pain Management of Osteoarthritis in the Human Knee Joint. *Aesthetic Surg. J.* **2016**, *36*, 229–236. [CrossRef]
16. Marx, R.E. Platelet-Rich Plasma (PRP): What Is PRP and What Is Not PRP? *Implant Dent.* **2001**, *10*, 225–228. [CrossRef]

17. Everts, P.; Onishi, K.; Jayaram, P.; Lana, J.F.; Mautner, K. Platelet-rich plasma: New performance understandings and therapeutic considerations in 2020. *Int. J. Mol. Sci.* **2020**, *21*, 7794. [CrossRef]
18. Mazzucco, L.; Balbo, V.; Cattana, E.; Guaschino, R.; Borzini, P. Not every PRP-gel is born equal Evaluation of growth factor availability for tissues through four PRP-gel preparations: Fibrinet®, RegenPRP-Kit®, Plateltex® and one manual procedure. *Vox Sang.* **2009**, *97*, 110–118. [CrossRef]
19. Degen, R.M.; Bernard, J.A.; Oliver, K.S.; Dines, J.S. Commercial Separation Systems Designed for Preparation of Platelet-Rich Plasma Yield Differences in Cellular Composition. *HSS J.* **2017**, *13*, 75–80. [CrossRef]
20. Wang, S.Z.; Rui, Y.F.; Tan, Q.; Wang, C. Enhancing intervertebral disc repair and regeneration through biology: Platelet-rich plasma as an alternative strategy. *Arthritis Res. Ther.* **2013**, *15*, 220. [CrossRef] [PubMed]
21. Knezevic, N.N.; Candido, K.D.; Desai, R.; Kaye, A.D. Is Platelet-Rich Plasma a Future Therapy in Pain Management? *Med. Clin. N. Am.* **2016**, *100*, 199–217. [CrossRef] [PubMed]
22. Migliorini, F.; Driessen, A.; Quack, V.; Sippel, N.; Cooper, B.; El Mansy, Y.; Tingart, M.; Eschweiler, J. Comparison between intra-articular infiltrations of placebo, steroids, hyaluronic and PRP for knee osteoarthritis: A Bayesian network meta-analysis. *Arch. Orthop. Trauma Surg.* **2021**, *141*, 1473–1490. [CrossRef]
23. Koh, Y.G.; Choi, Y.J. Infrapatellar fat pad-derived mesenchymal stem cell therapy for knee osteoarthritis. *Knee* **2012**, *19*, 902–907. [CrossRef] [PubMed]
24. Koh, Y.G.; Choi, Y.J.; Kwon, S.K.; Kim, Y.S.; Yeo, J.E. Clinical results and second-look arthroscopic findings after treatment with adipose-derived stem cells for knee osteoarthritis. *Knee Surg. Sport. Traumatol. Arthrosc.* **2015**, *23*, 1308–1316. [CrossRef] [PubMed]
25. Pak, J.; Chang, J.J.; Lee, J.H.; Lee, S.H. Safety reporting on implantation of autologous adipose tissue-derived stem cells with platelet-rich plasma into human articular joints. *BMC Musculoskelet. Disord.* **2013**, *14*, 337. [CrossRef] [PubMed]
26. Van Pham, P.; Bui, K.H.-T.; Duong, T.D.; Nguyen, N.T.; Nguyen, T.D.; Le, V.T.; Mai, V.T.; Phan, N.L.-C.; Le, D.M.; Ngoc, N.K. Symptomatic knee osteoarthritis treatment using autologous adipose derived stem cells and platelet-rich plasma: A clinical study. *Biomed. Res. Ther.* **2014**, *1*, 2–8. [CrossRef]
27. Bansal, H.; Comella, K.; Leon, J.; Verma, P.; Agrawal, D.; Koka, P.; Ichim, T. Intra-articular injection in the knee of adipose derived stromal cells (stromal vascular fraction) and platelet rich plasma for osteoarthritis. *J. Transl. Med.* **2017**, *15*, 141. [CrossRef]
28. Schouten, W.R.; Arkenbosch, J.H.C.; van der Woude, C.J.; de Vries, A.C.; Stevens, H.P.; Fuhler, G.M.; Dwarkasing, R.S.; van Ruler, O.; de Graaf, E.J.R. Efficacy and safety of autologous adipose-derived stromal vascular fraction enriched with platelet-rich plasma in flap repair of transsphincteric cryptoglandular fistulas. *Tech. Coloproctol.* **2021**, *25*, 1301–1309. [CrossRef]
29. DiMarino, A.M.; Caplan, A.I.; Bonfield, T.L. Mesenchymal Stem Cells in Tissue Repair. *Front. Immunol.* **2013**, *4*, 201. [CrossRef]
30. Molnar, V.; Pavelić, E.; Vrdoljak, K.; Čemerin, M.; Klarić, E.; Matišić, V.; Bjelica, R.; Brlek, P.; Kovačić, I.; Tremolada, C.; et al. Mesenchymal Stem Cell Mechanisms of Action and Clinical Effects in Osteoarthritis: A Narrative Review. *Genes* **2022**, *13*, 949. [CrossRef]
31. Baria, M.R.; Miller, M.M.; Borchers, J.; Desmond, S.; Onate, J.; Magnussen, R.; Vasileff, W.K.; Flanigan, D.; Kaeding, C.; Durgam, S. High Intensity Interval Exercise Increases Platelet and Transforming Growth Factor-β Yield in Platelet-Rich Plasma. *PM&R* **2020**, *12*, 1244–1250. [CrossRef]
32. Zenic, L.; Polancec, D.; Hudetz, D.; Jelec, Z.; Rod, E.; Vidovic, D.; Staresinic, M.; Sabalic, S.; Vrdoljak, T.; Petrovic, T.; et al. Polychromatic Flow Cytometric Analysis of Stromal Vascular Fraction from Lipoaspirate and Microfragmented Counterparts Reveals Sex-Related Immunophenotype Differences. *Genes* **2021**, *12*, 1999. [CrossRef] [PubMed]
33. Primorac, D.; Molnar, V.; Matišić, V.; Hudetz, D.; Jeleč, Ž.; Rod, E.; Čukelj, F.; Vidović, D.; Vrdoljak, T.; Dobričić, B.; et al. Comprehensive review of knee osteoarthritis pharmacological treatment and the latest professional societies' guidelines. *Pharmaceuticals* **2021**, *14*, 205. [CrossRef] [PubMed]
34. Kumar, A.; Kadamb, A.G.; Kadamb, K.G. Mesenchymal or maintenance stem cell & understanding their role in osteoarthritis of the knee joint: A review article. *Arch. Bone Jt. Surg.* **2020**, *8*, 560–569. [CrossRef] [PubMed]
35. Gupta, P.K.; Chullikana, A.; Rengasamy, M.; Shetty, N.; Pandey, V.; Agarwal, V.; Wagh, S.Y.; Vellotare, P.K.; Damodaran, D.; Viswanathan, P.; et al. Efficacy and safety of adult human bone marrow-derived, cultured, pooled, allogeneic mesenchymal stromal cells (Stempeucel®): Preclinical and clinical trial in osteoarthritis of the knee joint. *Arthritis Res. Ther.* **2016**, *18*, 301. [CrossRef]
36. Buzaboon, N.; Alshammary, S. Clinical Applicability of Adult Human Mesenchymal Stem Cell Therapy in the Treatment of Knee Osteoarthritis. *Stem Cells Cloning Adv. Appl.* **2020**, *13*, 117–136. [CrossRef]
37. Chahal, J.; Gómez-Aristizábal, A.; Shestopaloff, K.; Bhatt, S.; Chaboureau, A.; Fazio, A.; Chisholm, J.; Weston, A.; Chiovitti, J.; Keating, A.; et al. Bone Marrow Mesenchymal Stromal Cell Treatment in Patients with Osteoarthritis Results in Overall Improvement in Pain and Symptoms and Reduces Synovial Inflammation. *Stem Cells Transl. Med.* **2019**, *8*, 746–757. [CrossRef]
38. Crisan, M.; Yap, S.; Casteilla, L.; Chen, C.-W.; Corselli, M.; Park, T.S.; Andriolo, G.; Sun, B.; Zheng, B.; Zhang, L.; et al. A Perivascular Origin for Mesenchymal Stem Cells in Multiple Human Organs. *Cell Stem Cell* **2008**, *3*, 301–313. [CrossRef]
39. Su, X.; Wu, Z.; Chen, J.; Wu, N.; Ma, P.; Xia, Z.; Jiang, C.; Ye, Z.; Liu, S.; Liu, J.; et al. CD146 as a new marker for an increased chondroprogenitor cell sub-population in the later stages of osteoarthritis. *J. Orthop. Res.* **2015**, *33*, 84–91. [CrossRef]
40. Tremolada, C. Mesenchymal Stromal Cells and Micro Fragmented Adipose Tissue: New Horizons of Effectiveness of Lipogems. *J. Stem Cells Res. Dev. Ther.* **2019**, *5*, 017. [CrossRef]

41. Filardo, G.; Tschon, M.; Perdisa, F.; Brogini, S.; Cavallo, C.; Desando, G.; Giavaresi, G.; Grigolo, B.; Martini, L.; Nicoli Aldini, N.; et al. Micro-fragmentation is a valid alternative to cell expansion and enzymatic digestion of adipose tissue for the treatment of knee osteoarthritis: A comparative preclinical study. *Knee Surg. Sport. Traumatol. Arthrosc.* **2022**, *30*, 773–781. [CrossRef] [PubMed]
42. Michalek, J.; Moster, R.; Lukac, L.; Proefrock, K.; Petrasovic, M.; Rybar, J.; Chaloupka, A.; Darinskas, A.; Michalek, J.; Kristek, J.; et al. Stromal Vascular Fraction Cells of Adipose and Connective Tissue in People with Osteoarthritis: A Case Control Prospective Multi-Centric Non-Randomized Study. *Glob. Surg.* **2017**, *3*, 163. [CrossRef]
43. Belk, J.W.; Kraeutler, M.J.; Houck, D.A.; Goodrich, J.A.; Dragoo, J.L.; McCarty, E.C. Platelet-Rich Plasma Versus Hyaluronic Acid for Knee Osteoarthritis: A Systematic Review and Meta-analysis of Randomized Controlled Trials. *Am. J. Sport. Med.* **2021**, *49*, 249–260. [CrossRef] [PubMed]

Disclaimer/Publisher's Note: The statements, opinions and data contained in all publications are solely those of the individual author(s) and contributor(s) and not of MDPI and/or the editor(s). MDPI and/or the editor(s) disclaim responsibility for any injury to people or property resulting from any ideas, methods, instructions or products referred to in the content.

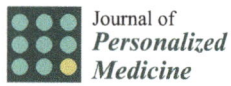

Article

Devascularized Bone Surface Culture: A Novel Strategy for Identifying Osteomyelitis-Related Pathogens

Peng Chen [1,2,3], Qing-rong Lin [1,2], Mou-Zhang Huang [1,4], Xin Zhang [1,5], Yan-jun Hu [1,2], Jing Chen [6], Nan Jiang [1,2,*] and Bin Yu [1,2,*]

1. Division of Orthopaedics & Traumatology, Department of Orthopaedics, Southern Medical University Nanfang Hospital, Guangzhou 510515, China
2. Guangdong Provincial Key Laboratory of Bone and Cartilage Regenerative Medicine, Southern Medical University Nanfang Hospital, Guangzhou 510515, China
3. Department of Orthopaedics, Hainan General Hospital, Hainan Hospital affiliated to Hainan Medical University, Haikou 570311, China
4. Department of Orthopaedics & Traumatology, Ganzhou Hospital Affiliated to Nanfang Hospital, Southern Medical University, Ganzhou 341099, China
5. Department of Orthopaedics, Wuyi Hospital of Traditional Chinese Medicine, Jiangmen 523000, China
6. Department of Laboratory Medicine, Southern Medical University Nanfang Hospital, Guangzhou 510515, China
* Correspondence: hnxyjn@smu.edu.cn (N.J.); yubin@smu.edu.cn (B.Y.); Tel.: +86-20-6278-6678 (N.J.); +86-20-6164-1741 (B.Y.)

Abstract: The gold standard for identifying pathogens causing osteomyelitis (OM) is intraoperative tissue sampling culture (TSC). However, its positive rate remains inadequate. Here, we evaluated the efficiency of a novel strategy, known as devitalized bone surface culture (BSC), for detecting OM-related microorganisms and compared it to TSC. Between December 2021 and July 2022, patients diagnosed with OM and received both methods for bacterial identification were screened for analysis. In total, 51 cases were finally recruited for analysis. The mean age was 43.6 years, with the tibia as the top infection site. The positive rate of BSC was relatively higher than that of TSC (74.5% vs. 58.8%, $p = 0.093$), though no statistical difference was achieved. Both BSC and TSC detected definite pathogens in 29 patients, and their results were in accordance with each other. The most frequent microorganism identified by the BSC method was *Staphylococcus aureus*. Moreover, BSC took a significantly shorter median culture time than TSC (1.0 days vs. 3.0 days, $p < 0.001$). In summary, BSC may be superior to TSC for identifying OM-associated pathogens, with a higher detectable rate and a shorter culture time.

Keywords: osteomyelitis; bone infection; bone surface culture; tissue sampling culture; *S. aureus*

Citation: Chen, P.; Lin, Q.-r.; Huang, M.-Z.; Zhang, X.; Hu, Y.-j.; Chen, J.; Jiang, N.; Yu, B. Devascularized Bone Surface Culture: A Novel Strategy for Identifying Osteomyelitis-Related Pathogens. *J. Pers. Med.* 2022, 12, 2050. https://doi.org/10.3390/jpm12122050

Academic Editor: Jih-Yang Ko

Received: 20 October 2022
Accepted: 8 December 2022
Published: 12 December 2022

Publisher's Note: MDPI stays neutral with regard to jurisdictional claims in published maps and institutional affiliations.

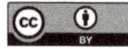

Copyright: © 2022 by the authors. Licensee MDPI, Basel, Switzerland. This article is an open access article distributed under the terms and conditions of the Creative Commons Attribution (CC BY) license (https://creativecommons.org/licenses/by/4.0/).

1. Introduction

Osteomyelitis (OM), also known as bone infection, is an inflammatory process following the invasion of pathogens, leading to inflammatory changes in osseous tissues [1]. It can occur following a contiguous focus, hematogenous spread, and vascular insufficiency [2]. Despite the great advances in the treatment, the clinical efficacy of OM remains inadequate, with an infection relapse rate ranging from 20% to 30% [3–5]. Such a high incidence of infection recurrence is associated with multiple factors [6], such as pathogen virulence, injury type, and treatment strategy.

The treatment of OM is complex and primarily depends on the initial causes and local pathological changes in patients [7]. Currently, treatment options include but are not limited to medullary space curettage, medullary reaming, medullary decompression, superficial decortication, sequestrectomy, soft tissue coverage, bone stabilization, and bone defect reconstruction [7]. Bone defects can be repaired by bone graft, Ilizarov technique, and Masquelet technique [1], or they may even be solved by utilizing bone tissue engineering strategies [8]. In addition to the aforementioned surgical interventions, one of the critical actions influencing the clinical efficacy of OM concerns antibiotic strategy, which is primarily on arthrocentesis and intraoperative sample cultures. Currently, standard intraoperative tissue sampling culture (TSC) is the gold standard for detecting the microorganisms which account for OM [9]. However, the positive rate of TSC remains inadequate, with most of the reported outcomes reaching around 60% [10]. Multiple factors affect its detectable rates, such as recent antibiotics and surgeries, the existence of bacteria biofilms, pathogen culture conditions, and sample selections [11]. Recently, different methods have been introduced and analyzed [10,12,13], aiming to increase the positive rate and guide the use of antibiotics.

In 2019, Moley and colleagues [14] reported using a novel method, the "agar candle dip", to map the biofilms on the orthopedic explants. Inspired by this approach, we introduced a new strategy for the bacterial detection of fracture implant-associated infections (IAIs), known as "implant surface culture" (ISC) [15], based on the hypothesis that implant surfaces may be attached to bacterial biofilms. The outcomes of 42 patients demonstrated that the positive rate of ISC was significantly higher than that of TSC (85.7% vs. 54.8%, $p = 0.002$), signaling the definite efficiency of such a method as an adjunct treatment for bacterial identification purposes. Nonetheless, as mentioned in this study [15], one limitation is that it cannot be performed in the case of the retention of the implant hardware. In addition, there are still many OM patients without implants; thus, avenues to improve the detectable rate in such a group of patients require further exploration.

It is established that one of the typical histological characteristics of OM is the existence or formation of devascularized bone with or without sequestrum, which may provide a function for the attachment of bacteria biofilms [16], similar to those attached to the implants. Thus, we hypothesized that the direct culture on such object surfaces, referred to as "bone surface culture" (BSC), may increase the positive rate. Here, we compared the efficiency of BSC with TSC to detect OM-related microorganisms.

2. Materials and Methods

2.1. Study Setting, OM Diagnostic Criteria, and Inclusion and Exclusion Criteria

This prospective study was performed at Southern Medical University Nanfang Hospital, a tertiary medical center in Guangzhou, South China. The diagnosis of OM was referred to the diagnostic criteria of fracture-related infection (FRI) [17,18], including a sinus tract or fistula, wound breakdown or pus directly connecting the bone, visible pathogens measured via the histological test, and over five neutrophils per high power field (NP/HPF) [19]. The patients included were those with a confirmed diagnosis of OM following a contiguous focus or hematogenous spread, those with signed informed consent, those who stopped antibiotic use for at least two weeks, and those who received both methods for pathogen identification purposes. Patients were excluded if they were diagnosed with vascular insufficiency-related OM, joint infections, and prosthetic joint infections (PJIs) or received conservative treatment. In addition, patient data with any violations against prespecified BSC or TSC protocols were excluded. This study was conducted in line with the tenets of the 1964 Helsinki declaration and was approved by the Medical Ethical Committee of the Southern Medical University Nanfang Hospital (NFEC-2020-075).

2.2. BSC and TSC Procedures

All the included patients had stopped taking antibiotics for at least two weeks before surgery commenced. Intraoperative intravenous cephalosporins or clindamycin were administered only after the specimens were collected for culture and histology purposes. The same experienced surgeon collected the samples for both BSC and TSC.

The BSC procedure was similar to that of ISC [15]. First, the devascularized bone fragments, collected as much as possible, were directly set in an aseptic culture plate with congealed tryptic soy agar (TSA) at the bottom of the operation room. Then, the culture plate was transported to the biosafety cabinet of the laboratory within two hours.

Then, the surface of the osseous tissue was gently covered with cooled and molten TSA. After that, the plate was incubated at 37 °C with 5% CO_2. Sterile TSA was carefully added when necessary, to prevent the surfaces from drying out. The surfaces of the bone tissues and their surrounding culture media were examined every day for two weeks, as recommended [20], or until the colonies of the microorganisms appeared. If colonies were found, three different sites of colonies were separately swabbed and inoculated into the blood culture bottles. Then, the colonies were sampled by inoculating loops, and a mass spectrometer (Biomerieux, VITEK MS, Marcy-l'Étoile, France) was used for bacterial identification. A schematic diagram of the BSC procedure is depicted in Figure 1.

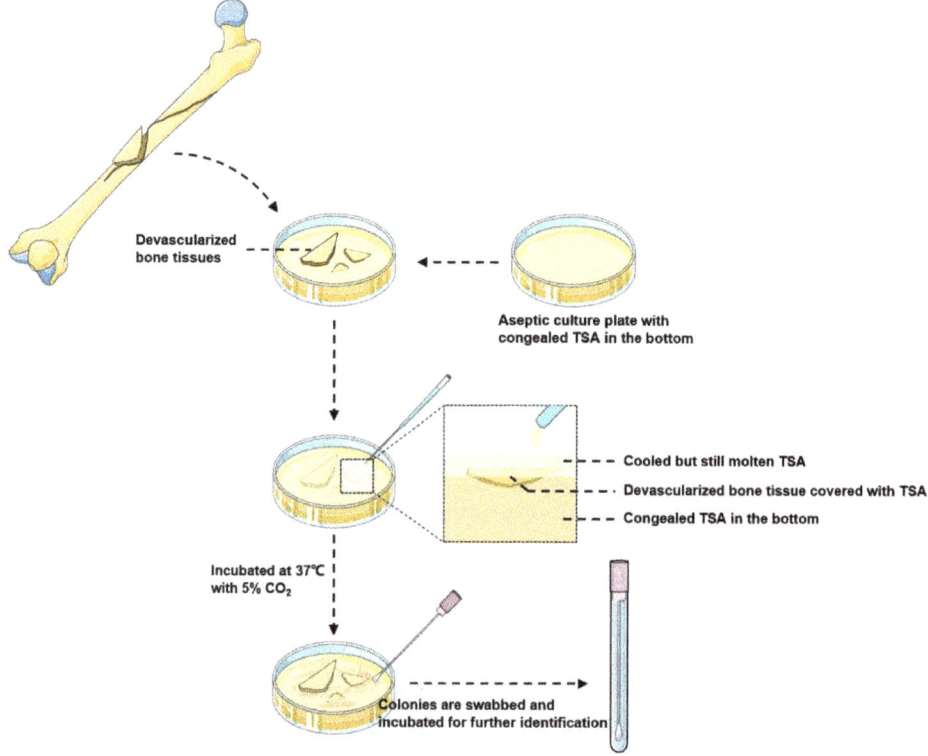

Figure 1. The schematic diagram of the BSC procedure.

For TSC, the specimens from five different sites that were highly suspected of OM were collected. Then, the samples were disposed of by the working staff of the Clinical Laboratory within two hours. First, normal saline (10 mL) was used to homogenize the specimens separately with glass beads. Then, they were inoculated into the blood culture bottles (the BACTEC Lytic/10 Anaerobic/F bottle and the BACTEC Plus Aerobic/F bottle, Becton, Dickinson and Company, MD, Franklin Lakes, NJ, USA). The bottles were incubated at 37 °C with 5% CO_2 for at least one week. Similarly, any identified colonies were collected by inoculating loops using the mass spectrometer (Biomerieux, VITEK MS, Marcy-l'Étoile, France) for bacterial identification purposes.

2.3. Statistical Analysis

The Statistical Package for Social Sciences software (version 17.0, SPSS Inc., Chicago, IL, USA) was used to conduct statistical analysis. The chi-square test was used to compare the positive rate, and a Wilcoxon signed-rank test was applied to compare the culture time, between the two methods. Statistical significance was defined as a p-value of ≤ 0.05.

3. Results

3.1. Participant Inclusion Flow Chart, Patient Demographics, OM Etiology, Body Side, and Infection Site Distributions

A total of 67 patients were initially screened. After applying the inclusion and exclusion criteria, 51 patients (43 males) were finally included. A flow chart is depicted in Figure 2. The mean age of the included patients at diagnosis was 43.6 ± 17.4 years, with mean ages of 42.8 ± 17.0 years and 48.4 ± 20.0 years for males and females, respectively (p = 0.408). Among the 51 OM patients, 42 were classified as post-traumatic OM, with nine classified as hematogenous spread-related infection. Infections on the right body side were found in 26 cases, with 25 on the left side. The top three infected sites were the tibia (25 cases), calcaneus (11 cases), and femur (8 cases), followed by the humerus (3 cases), toes (2 cases), radius (1 case), and ulna (1 case) (Table 1).

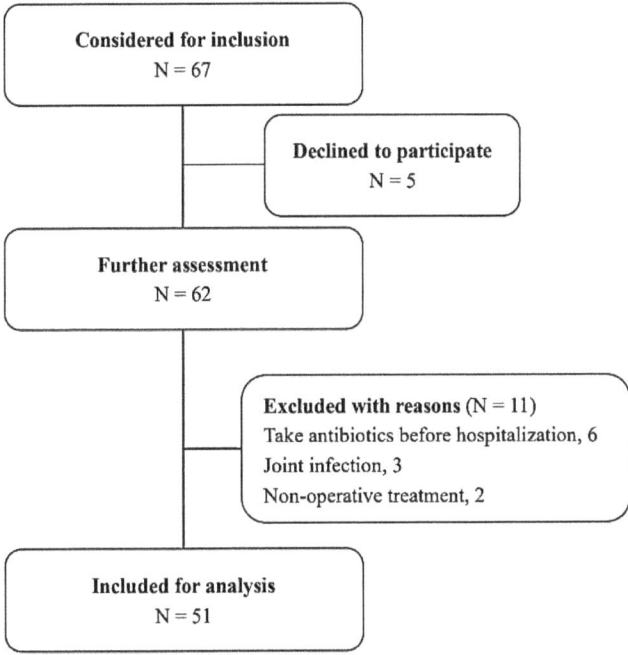

Figure 2. Eligibility selection process of the OM patients in this study.

Table 1. Clinical features of the included OM patients, culture outcomes, and culture time by BSC and TSC.

Case No.	Sex/Age (Year)	Infection Site	BSC Outcome	BSC Time (Day)	TSC Outcome	TSC Time (Day)
1	M/14	Femur	*Staphylococcus aureus*	1	*Staphylococcus aureus*	3
2	M/29	Tibia	*Staphylococcus aureus*	1	*Staphylococcus aureus*	3
3	M/41	Tibia	*Achromobacter xylosoxidans* + *Acinetobacter lwoffii*	3	Negative	NA
4	M/49	Tibia	*Escherichia coli*	1	*Escherichia coli*	3
5	F/49	Calcaneus	Negative	NA	Negative	NA
6	M/44	Tibia	*Staphylococcus epidermidis*	3	Negative	NA
7	M/53	Femur	*Staphylococcus aureus*	1	*Staphylococcus aureus*	3
8	M/14	Tibia	*Streptococcus pyogenes*	1	*Streptococcus pyogenes*	2
9	F/32	Tibia	*Candida parapsilosis*	1	*Candida parapsilosis*	2

Table 1. Cont.

Case No.	Sex/Age (Year)	Infection Site	BSC Outcome	BSC Time (Day)	TSC Outcome	TSC Time (Day)
10	M/71	Tibia	Proteus mirabilis	1	Proteus mirabilis	2
11	M/59	Femur	Proteus mirabilis	1	Proteus mirabilis	2
12	M/10	Phalange	Staphylococcus epidermidis	1	Staphylococcus epidermidis	3
13	M/53	Calcaneus	Proteus mirabilis + Staphylococcus felis	1	Proteus mirabilis + Staphylococcus felis	5
14	M/51	Calcaneus	Staphylococcus aureus	1	Staphylococcus aureus	4
15	M/59	Radius	Staphylococcus aureus	1	Negative	NA
16	M/21	Humerus	Negative	NA	Negative	NA
17	M/50	Tibia	Staphylococcus aureus	1	Staphylococcus aureus	2
18	M/49	Tibia	Staphylococcus aureus	1	Staphylococcus aureus	4
19	M/16	Femur	Enterococcus faecalis	1	Negative	NA
20	F/68	Tibia	Negative	NA	Negative	NA
21	M/68	Calcaneus	Proteus mirabilis	1	Proteus mirabilis	3
22	F/54	Calcaneus	Negative	NA	Negative	NA
23	M/46	Calcaneus	Staphylococcus aureus	1	Staphylococcus aureus	3
24	F/48	Femur	Staphylococcus aureus	1	Staphylococcus aureus	4
25	M/42	Tibia	Enterobacter cloacae	1	Negative	NA
26	M/37	Tibia	Negative	NA	Negative	NA
27	M/39	Tibia	Mycobacterium fortuitum	3	Mycobacterium fortuitum	3
28	M/87	Humerus	Pseudomonas aeruginosa	3	Pseudomonas aeruginosa	3
29	M/52	Calcaneus	Negative	NA	Negative	NA
30	M/47	Calcaneus	Staphylococcus aureus	1	Staphylococcus aureus	3
31	M/15	Tibia	Negative	NA	Negative	NA
32	M/29	Phalange	Staphylococcus aureus	1	Staphylococcus aureus	2
33	M/36	Femur	Negative	NA	Staphylococcus aureus	3
34	M/52	Tibia	Pseudomonas aeruginosa	3	Negative	NA
35	M/56	Tibia	Staphylococcus warneri	2	Staphylococcus warneri	3
36	M/32	Tibia	Negative	NA	Negative	NA
37	M/67	Calcaneus	Escherichia coli	1	Escherichia coli	4
38	M/29	Tibia	Staphylococcus haemolyticus	1	Staphylococcus haemolyticus	3
39	M/45	Calcaneus	Negative	NA	Negative	NA
40	M/37	Tibia	Negative	NA	Negative	NA
41	M/49	Ulna	Serratia marcescens	1	Negative	NA
42	M/66	Tibia	Staphylococcus aureus	1	Staphylococcus aureus	2
43	M/25	Tibia	Staphylococcus aureus	1	Staphylococcus aureus	3
44	M/48	Calcaneus	Streptococcus agalactiae	1	Streptococcus agalactiae	4
45	F/63	Tibia	Streptococcus dysgalactiae	2	Streptococcus dysgalactiae	3
46	M/30	Tibia	Proteus mirabilis	1	Negative	NA
47	M/43	Femur	Enterobacter aerogenes	1	Enterobacter aerogenes	3
48	M/49	Tibia	Negative	NA	Negative	NA
49	F/8	Tibia	Negative	NA	Negative	NA
50	M/30	Femur	Escherichia coli + Enterococcus	1	Escherichia coli + Enterococcus	2
51	F/65	Humerus	Enterobacter asburiae + Enterococcus faecalis	2	Negative	NA

OM: osteomyelitis; BSC: Bone surface culture; TSC: tissue sampling culture; NA: not available.

3.2. BSC and TSC Outcomes and Culture Time

The total positive rate of BSC (38/51) was relatively higher than TSC (30/51), though no statistical difference was found (74.5% vs. 58.8%, $p = 0.093$). Both BSC and TSC detected definite pathogens in 29 patients, and their results were in accordance with each other. In addition, BSC took a significantly shorter median culture time than TSC (1.0 days vs. 3.0 days, $p < 0.001$). The graphical representation of the primary outcomes of the present study is depicted in Figure 3. The detailed results regarding both of the methods are presented in Table 1. Figure 4 shows nine patients with positive outcomes, whereas Figure 5 displays three patients with negative outcomes, measured via the BSC method.

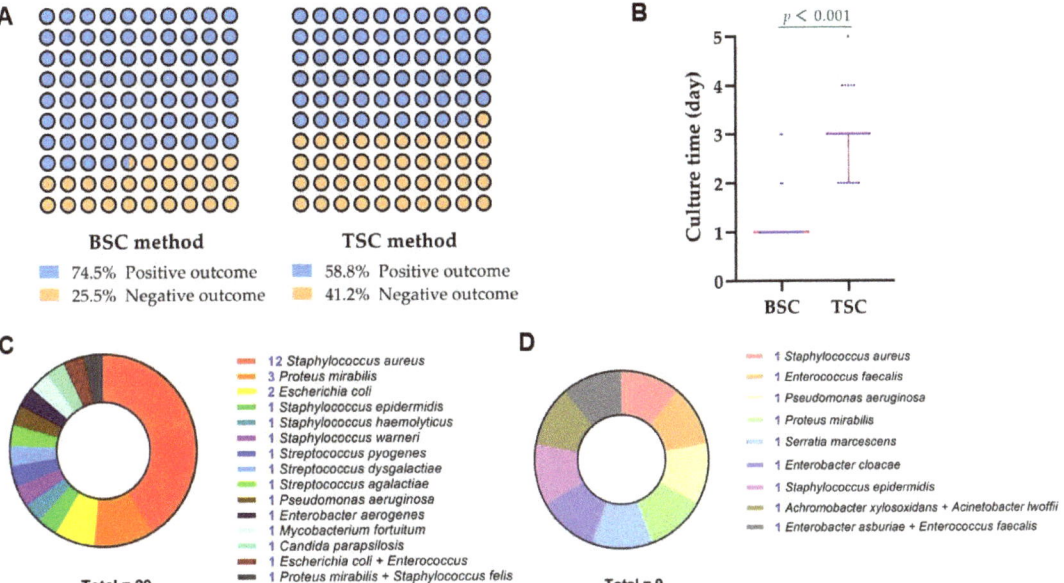

Figure 3. Graphical representation of the primary outcomes of the current study. Panel (**A**): Positive rates of the BSC and TSC strategies. Panel (**B**): The culture time of the BSC group was shorter than TSC group (a Wilcoxon signed-rank test, $p < 0.001$). Panel (**C**): Distribution of the microorganisms detected by both BSC and TSC, with consistent results. Panel (**D**): Distribution of the microorganisms identified by only BSC while TSC showed negative outcomes.

3.3. Microorganism Type

The BSC method detected 38 patients with definite pathogens, and 34 were identified as having monomicrobial infections. The most frequent pathogen was *Staphylococcus aureus* (13 cases), followed by *Proteus mirabilis* (4 cases), *Pseudomonas aeruginosa* (2 cases), *Escherichia coli* (2 cases), and *Staphylococcus epidermidis* (2 cases). Another 11 types of microorganisms were only found in a single patient (Table 1), including a fungus, *Candida parapsilosis*.

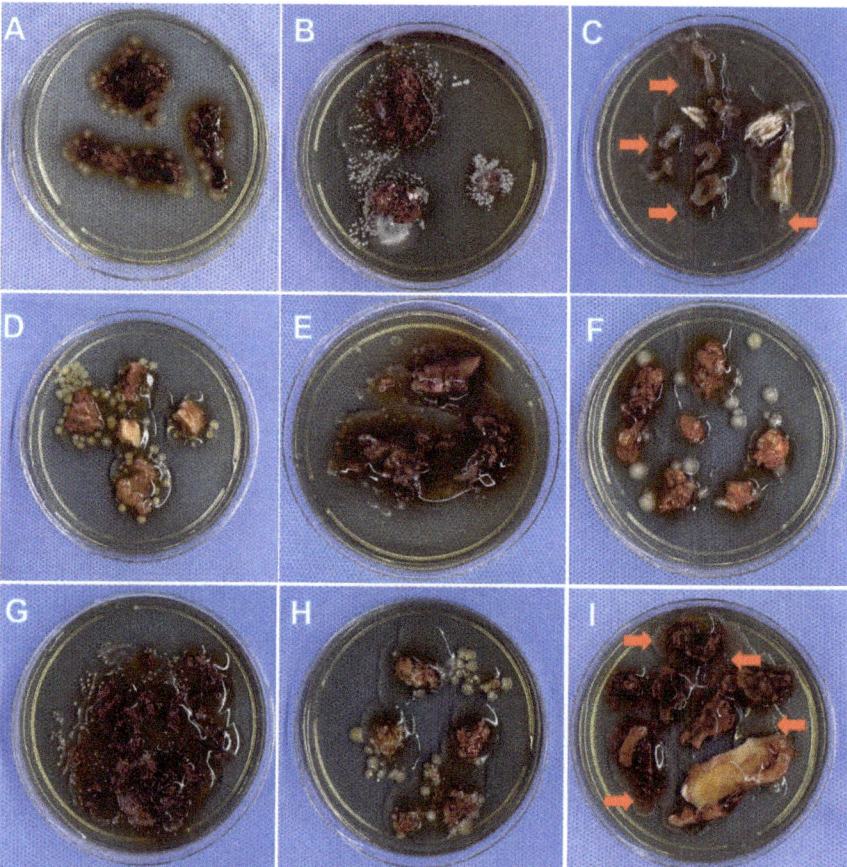

Figure 4. Nine OM patients showed positive outcomes using the BSC method. Panel (**A**): 49-year-old, male, tibia OM, BSC: *Escherichia coli*, TSC: *Escherichia coli*. Panel (**B**): 32-year-old, female, BSC: *Candida parapsilosis*, TSC: *Candida parapsilosis*. Panel (**C**): 71-year-old, male, tibia OM, BSC: *Proteus mirabilis*, TSC: *Proteus mirabilis* (see the arrows). Panel (**D**): 50-year-old, male, tibial OM, BSC: *Staphylococcus aureus*, TSC: *Staphylococcus aureus*. Panel (**E**): 16-year-old, male, femoral OM, BSC: *Enterococcus faecalis*, TSC: Negative. Panel (**F**): 42-year-old, male, tibia OM, BSC: *Enterobacter cloacae*, TSC: Negative. Panel (**G**): 39-year-old, male, tibia OM, BSC: *Mycobacterium fortuitum*, TSC: *Mycobacterium fortuitum*. Panel (**H**): 47-year-old, male, calcaneal OM, BSC: *Staphylococcus aureus*, TSC: *Staphylococcus aureus*. Panel (**I**): 43-year-old, male, femoral OM, BSC: *Enterobacter aerogenes*, TSC: *Enterobacter aerogenes* (see the arrows).

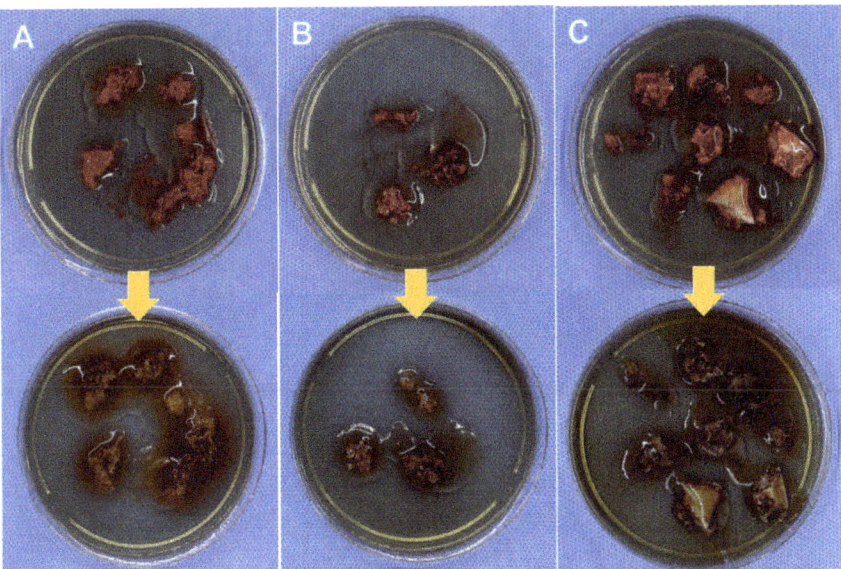

Figure 5. Three OM patients revealed negative outcomes by the BSC method (images in the upper row: the initial stage of BSC; images in the lower row: the end stage of BSC). Panel (**A**): 15-year-old, male, tibia OM, TSC: negative. Panel (**B**): 32-year-old, male, tibia OM, TSC: negative. Panel (**C**): 37-year-old, male, tibia OM, TSC: negative.

4. Discussion

As mentioned previously, aside from surgery, the timely, effective, and correct identification of OM-related pathogens is one of the most critical measures that can be taken to decrease the risk of infection recurrence and improve treatment efficacy. However, currently, the efficiency of TSC remains inadequate. According to a recent multicenter study in Northeast China [21], the positive rate of traditional culture among FRI patients was only 50.8%, which is far from satisfying. To increase the detection rate, several novel strategies of culture have been reported and analyzed, such as sonication fluid culture [12] and culture from the reamer–irrigator–aspirator (RIA) system [13]. In a prospective cohort study, Finelli et al. [12] compared the efficiency between traditional peri-implant tissue culture and sonication fluid culture in patients with intramedullary nailing infection. The outcomes of 54 patients revealed that the positive rates of conventional culture and sonication fluid culture were similar (89.4% vs. 97.6%), while the sonication fluid culture displayed advantages in identifying polymicrobial infections. In addition to the sonication fluid culture, Onsea et al. [13] introduced a strategy of cultures from the RIA system. The results from 24 patients indicate that such a novel method displayed similar efficiency when compared to the standard tissue culture (71% vs. 67%). The current BSC method also revealed similar diagnostic accuracy with the RIA system culture (74.5% vs. 71%) but was inferior to the sonication fluid culture. Nonetheless, all three novel strategies had advantages over TSC.

Recently, Moley et al. [14] reported using an "agar candle dip" method to map biofilms on orthopedic explants. In light of this study, we tried to cover the culture medium on the surfaces of the explants among patients with IAIs and achieved satisfactory outcomes [15]. However, one intrinsic limitation of this method is that it cannot be conducted among patients without implants, which limits its application. Here, we expanded and modified this method and directly poured TSA on the devascularized bone surface, which resembled an implant surface, where many great biofilms might also become attached. Outcomes demonstrated that the delay of positivity was hugely reduced with the BSC method compared to TSC, suggesting that BSC is also a valuable approach for detecting OM-related pathogens, especially those without implants. We believe that one primary reason accounting for the superiority of BSC over TSC is that all the available devascularized bone tissues are collected and cultured, lowering the risk of selection bias to the minimum.

Although the current BSC strategy is referred to as the "agar candle dip" method, the efficiency of BSC appears to be superior. It can be primarily attributed to several possible factors. First, Moley and colleagues used different types of materials from the prosthesis for culture purposes, while we only cultured the devascularized bone tissue. Secondly, they used brain heart infusion (BHI) agar, whereas we used TSA agar. The case of whether the culture medium influences the detection efficiency requires further investigation. Thirdly, Moley et al. incubated the components for seven days, while we extended such a culture time to 14 days. Of course, the decision regarding whether 14-day incubation is necessary needs to be evaluated in the future. Lastly, they included only 15 patients for analysis, which may also affect the outcomes.

The present BSC technique shares similarities and differences with ISC. For similarities, firstly, both BSC and ISC used the same culture medium, TSA, to cover the in vitro tissues and implants. As one of the most frequently used culture media, TSA acts as a general-purpose non-selective medium providing abundant nutrients which allow a wide variety of microorganisms to grow and can also be used for the storage, maintenance, and transportation of pure pathogens. However, the case of whether TSA is the optimal medium requires further analysis. Secondly, the culture conditions and duration of the two methods are the same, both with incubation at 37 °C under 5% CO_2, with a consecutive run of 14 days or until the appearance of colonies of the microorganisms. Third, as both of the methods require TSA agar supplementation during culture, repeated exposures of the tissues or implants increase the contamination risk. Therefore, on the one hand, necessary controls should be set to identify whether contaminations occur or not clearly. On the other hand, procedures and tools may be modified to lower such risks to the minimum.

Regarding differences, firstly, we did not rinse the devascularized bone tissues with normal saline before culture, as we would like to keep the original situation or status of the deep tissues and lower the contamination risk. The case of whether rinsing is an essential procedure for BSC needs further exploration. Secondly, our study was different from ISC as there was nothing on the bottom of the culture plate. Meanwhile, for BSC, already congealed TSA was prepared in advance in the bottom before the osseous tissues were placed. The primary reason is that, quite different from explants; the bone tissues may lose vitality and quickly become dry without the medium in the bottom. Thirdly, BSC may display a higher risk of selection bias than ISC. For ISC, the whole implants are obtained and covered with TSA. Whereas the selection of devascularized bone tissues largely relies on the surgeons' experiences with BSC, though the specimens have been selected and cultured as much as possible, selection bias cannot be avoided entirely. Further within-person comparisons should be conducted to evaluate the efficacy levels between BSC and ISC.

Interestingly, *Candida parapsilosis* was found by BSC in a 32-year-old female patient with OM following trauma, and the TSC result also confirmed such a type of fungi. Fungal OM and septic arthritis are rare, with *Candida* and *Aspergillus* being the most frequent agents [22]. In 2016, Gamaletsou et al. [23] summarized the clinical features, diagnosis, and treatment of *Candida*-related arthritis based on the synthesis of reported cases within the literature. The outcomes of 112 patients demonstrated that *Candida*-related arthritis primarily affects the hips and the knees. Despite antifungal therapy, the successful treatment of such an infection still poses significant challenges. In addition to the case of fungi-related infection, *Mycobacterium fortuitum* was detected by both methods in a 39-year-old male diagnosed with tibia OM. It is known that *Mycobacterium fortuitum* is a type of slow-growing bacterium which is often associated with contamination. OM related to *Mycobacterium fortuitum* is rare and was occasionally presented as a single case report. In 2015, Grantham et al. [24] reported OM related to *Mycobacterium fortuitum* in a 14-year-old patient following reconstruction surgery for the anterior cruciate ligament. The infection was successfully eradicated by repeated debridement and irrigation with systematic and local antibiotics. Recently, Fraga et al. [25] also presented a case diagnosed of OM associated with *Mycobacterium fortuitum* in the cuboid bone of a 61-year-old female. She was successfully treated by debridement in combination with the local implantation of calcium sulfate containing gentamicin and vancomycin.

It is also notable that one patient showed a negative result following BSC, while TSC showed infection associated with *S. aureus*. Such an unexpected result may be correlated with selection bias during sample collections. To further increase the detection rate, integrated and standardized sampling procedures for BSC should be established. Aside from sample selections, another factor that may lead to negative results is that both BSC and ISC cannot identify the anaerobic bacteria associated with the intrinsic limitation of the two strategies. In this study, we excluded patients with OM related to vascular insufficiency (e.g., diabetic foot OM), mainly because most of these patients usually have ulcers which may increase the risk of contamination.

In addition to the above-mentioned intrinsic limitations of the BSC method, our study also has several limitations. Firstly, the method reported in this paper is preliminary and requires further optimization. Moreover, the sample dispensing and culture strategy indeed have significant room for refinement and improvement. To better evaluate the efficiency of this novel strategy, a well-designed study with a larger sample size as well as necessary controls is warranted to calculate the sensitivity, specificity, and diagnostic accuracy of OM. Secondly, this study did not analyze the risk factors linked to the negative outcomes of BSC, which need to be further investigated. Thirdly, although both BSC and ISC have shown satisfying results, the better of the two remains to be seen as their direct comparisons are lacking. Fourthly, we did not assess therapeutic efficacy as the follow-up time was short. Thus, future studies should focus on the treatment efficacy and its potential influencing factors.

5. Conclusions

In conclusion, our study suggests that BSC may be an effective and valuable strategy for identifying microorganisms that cause OM, with a higher positive rate and a shorter culture time. Procedures of this method should be optimized to increase the detection rate of OM-related pathogens.

Author Contributions: P.C. and Q.-r.L. contributed equally to this study. Conceptualization, N.J. and B.Y.; methodology, P.C., Q.-r.L., Y.-j.H. and J.C.; formal analysis, X.Z., N.J. and B.Y.; investigation, P.C., Q.-r.L., M.-Z.H., X.Z., Y.-j.H. and J.C.; writing—original draft preparation, P.C.; writing—review and editing, N.J. and B.Y.; supervision, N.J.; project administration, N.J. and B.Y.; funding acquisition, N.J. and B.Y. All authors have read and agreed to the published version of the manuscript.

Funding: This research was funded by the National Natural Science Foundation of China (grant numbers: 82172197, 82272517) and Guangdong Basic and Applied Basic Research Foundation (grant number: 2022A1515012385).

Institutional Review Board Statement: The study was approved by the Medical Ethical Committee of Southern Medical University Nanfang Hospital (Approval number: NFEC-2020-075).

Informed Consent Statement: Informed consent was obtained from all subjects involved in the study. Written informed consent has been obtained from the patients to publish this paper.

Data Availability Statement: Not applicable.

Acknowledgments: The authors would like to thank Lei Fan, from the Division of Joint Surgery, Department of Orthopaedics, Southern Medical University Nanfang Hospital, for his help in drawing the schematic diagram of the BSC procedure.

Conflicts of Interest: The authors declare no conflict of interest.

References

1. Arshad, Z.; Lau, E.J.-S.; Aslam, A.; Thahir, A.; Krkovic, M. Management of chronic osteomyelitis of the femur and tibia: A scoping review. *EFORT Open Rev.* **2021**, *6*, 704–715. [CrossRef] [PubMed]
2. Lew, D.P.; Waldvogel, F.A. Osteomyelitis. *Lancet* **2004**, *364*, 369–379. [CrossRef] [PubMed]
3. Panteli, M.; Giannoudis, P.V. Chronic osteomyelitis: What the surgeon needs to know. *EFORT Open Rev.* **2016**, *1*, 128–135. [CrossRef] [PubMed]
4. Mathews, J.; Ward, J.; Chapman, T.; Khan, U.; Kelly, M. Single-stage orthoplastic reconstruction of Gustilo–Anderson Grade III open tibial fractures greatly reduces infection rates. *Injury* **2015**, *46*, 2263–2266. [CrossRef] [PubMed]
5. Lazzarini, L.; Mader, J.T.; Calhoun, J.H. Osteomyelitis in long bones. *J. Bone Joint Surg. Am.* **2004**, *86*, 2305–2318. [CrossRef]
6. Yong, T.M.; Rackard, F.A.; Dutton, L.K.; Sparks, M.B.; Harris, M.B.; Gitajn, I.L. Analyzing risk factors for treatment failure in fracture-related infection. *Arch. Orthop. Trauma Surg.* **2022**. [CrossRef]
7. Birt, M.C.; Anderson, D.W.; Toby, E.B.; Wang, J. Osteomyelitis: Recent advances in pathophysiology and therapeutic strategies. *J. Orthop.* **2017**, *14*, 45–52. [CrossRef]
8. Pardo, A.; Gómez-Florit, M.; Barbosa, S.; Taboada, P.; Domingues, R.M.A.; Gomes, M.E. Magnetic Nanocomposite Hydrogels for Tissue Engineering: Design Concepts and Remote Actuation Strategies to Control Cell Fate. *ACS Nano* **2021**, *15*, 175–209. [CrossRef]
9. Post, J.C.; A Preston, R.; Aul, J.J.; Larkins-Pettigrew, M.; Rydquist-White, J.; Anderson, K.W.; Wadowsky, R.M.; Reagan, D.R.; Walker, E.S.; A Kingsley, L.; et al. Molecular analysis of bacterial pathogens in otitis media with effusion. *JAMA* **1995**, *273*, 1598–1604. [CrossRef]
10. Ahmed, E.A.; Almutairi, M.K.; Alkaseb, A.T. Accuracy of Tissue and Sonication Fluid Sampling for the Diagnosis of Fracture-Related Infection: Diagnostic Meta-Analysis. *Cureus* **2021**, *13*, e14925. [CrossRef]
11. Dudareva, M.; Barrett, L.; Morgenstern, M.; Atkins, B.; Brent, A.; McNally, M. Providing an Evidence Base for Tissue Sampling and Culture Interpretation in Suspected Fracture-Related Infection. *J. Bone Joint Surg. Am.* **2021**, *103*, 977–983. [CrossRef] [PubMed]
12. Finelli, C.A.; da Silva, C.B.; Murça, M.A.; dos Reis, F.B.; Miki, N.; Fernandes, H.A.; Dell'Aquila, A.; Salles, M.J. Microbiological diagnosis of intramedullary nailing infection: Comparison of bacterial growth between tissue sampling and sonication fluid cultures. *Int. Orthop.* **2021**, *45*, 565–573. [CrossRef] [PubMed]
13. Onsea, J.; Pallay, J.; Depypere, M.; Moriarty, T.F.; Van Lieshout, E.M.; Obremskey, W.T.; Sermon, A.; Hoekstra, H.; Verhofstad, M.H.; Nijs, S.; et al. Intramedullary tissue cultures from the Reamer-Irrigator-Aspirator system for diagnosing fracture-related infection. *J. Orthop. Res.* **2020**, *39*, 281–290. [CrossRef] [PubMed]
14. Moley, J.P.; McGrath, M.S.; Granger, J.F.; Sullivan, A.C.; Stoodley, P.; Dusane, D. Mapping bacterial biofilms on recovered orthopaedic implants by a novel agar candle dip method. *APMIS* **2019**, *127*, 123–130. [CrossRef] [PubMed]
15. Liang, N.; Hu, Y.J.; Lin, Q.R.; Chen, P.; Wan, H.Y.; He, S.Y.; Stoodley, P.; Yu, B. Implant surface culture may be a useful adjunct to standard tissue sampling culture for identification of pathogens accounting for fracture-device-related infection: A within-person randomized agreement study of 42 patients. *Acta Orthop.* **2022**, *93*, 703–708.
16. Hofstee, M.I.; Muthukrishnan, G.; Atkins, G.J.; Riool, M.; Thompson, K.; Morgenstern, M.; Stoddart, M.J.; Richards, R.G.; Zaat, S.A.J.; Moriarty, T.F. Current Concepts of Osteomyelitis: From Pathologic Mechanisms to Advanced Research Methods. *Am. J. Pathol* **2020**, *190*, 1151–1163. [CrossRef]
17. McNally, M.; Govaert, G.; Dudareva, M.; Morgenstern, M.; Metsemakers, W.-J. Definition and diagnosis of fracture-related infection. *EFORT Open Rev.* **2020**, *5*, 614–619. [CrossRef]
18. Govaert, G.A.M.; Kuehl, R.; Atkins, B.L.; Trampuz, A.; Morgenstern, M.; Obremskey, W.T.; Verhofstad, M.H.J.; McNally, M.A.; Metsemakers, W.-J. Diagnosing Fracture-Related Infection: Current Concepts and Recommendations. *J. Orthop. Trauma* **2020**, *34*, 8–17. [CrossRef]
19. Morgenstern, M.; Athanasou, N.A.; Ferguson, J.Y.; Metsemakers, W.-J.; Atkins, B.L.; McNally, M.A. The value of quantitative histology in the diagnosis of fracture-related infection. *Bone Joint J.* **2018**, *100*, 966–972. [CrossRef]
20. Steinmetz, S.; Wernly, D.; Moerenhout, K.; Trampuz, A.; Borens, O. Infection after fracture fixation. *EFORT Open Rev.* **2019**, *4*, 468–475. [CrossRef]
21. Wang, B.; Xiao, X.; Zhang, J.; Han, W.; Hersi, S.A.; Tang, X. Epidemiology and microbiology of fracture-related infection: A multicenter study in Northeast China. *J. Orthop. Surg. Res.* **2021**, *16*, 490. [CrossRef] [PubMed]
22. Bariteau, J.T.; Waryasz, G.R.; McDonnell, M.; Fischer, S.A.; Hayda, C.R.A.; Born, C.T. Fungal osteomyelitis and Septic Arthritis. *J. Am. Acad. Orthop. Surg.* **2014**, *22*, 390–401. [CrossRef] [PubMed]
23. Gamaletsou, M.N.; Rammaert, B.; Bueno, M.A.; Sipsas, N.V.; Moriyama, B.; Kontoyiannis, D.P.; Roilides, E.; Zeller, V.; Taj-Aldeen, S.J.; Miller, A.O.; et al. Candida Arthritis: Analysis of 112 Pediatric and Adult Cases. *Open Forum Infect. Dis.* **2015**, *3*, ofv207. [CrossRef] [PubMed]
24. Grantham, W.J.; Raynor, M.B.; Martus, J.E. Articular Sinus Tract with Mycobacterium fortuitum Osteomyelitis After Anterior Cruciate Ligament Reconstruction: A Case Report. *JBJS Case Connect.* **2015**, *5*, e105. [CrossRef] [PubMed]
25. Fraga, K.; Maireles, M.; Jordan, M.; Soldevila, L.; Murillo, O. *Mycobacterium fortuitum* osteomyelitis of the cuboid bone treated with CERAMENT G and V: A case report. *JBJT* **2022**, *7*, 163–167. [CrossRef] [PubMed]

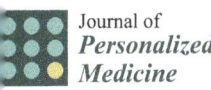

Article

Which Is Better in Clinical and Radiological Outcomes for Lumbar Degenerative Disease of Two Segments: MIS-TLIF or OPEN-TLIF?

Weiran Hu [1,†], Guang Yang [1,†], Hongqiang Wang [1], Xiaonan Wu [2], Haohao Ma [1], Kai Zhang [1] and Yanzheng Gao [1,*]

1 Department of Spine and Spinal Cord Surgery, People's Hospital of Zhengzhou University, Zhengzhou 450003, China
2 Department of Spine and Spinal Cord Surgery, People's Hospital of Henan University, Zhengzhou 450003, China
* Correspondence: gaoyanzhengspine@163.com
† These authors contributed equally to this work.

Abstract: Objective: To compare the clinical and radiological outcomes of minimally invasive transforaminal lumbar interbody fusion (MIS-TLIF) and traditional open transforaminal lumbar interbody fusion (OPEN-TLIF) in the treatment of two-level lumbar degenerative diseases. Methods: The clinical data of 112 patients were retrospectively analyzed, and were divided into an MIS-TLIF group and OPEN-TLIF group. The operative time, intraoperative fluoroscopy, blood loss, postoperative drainage volume, bed rest time, the content of creatine kinase(CK) and complications, were recorded. VAS score and ODI index were used to evaluate clinical efficacy. Bridwell grading was used to evaluate postoperative interbody fusion. Screw position was evaluated by Rao grading. Results: Compared with the OPEN-TLIF group, the MIS-TLIF group had longer operation times, more intraoperative fluoroscopy times, but shorter postoperative bed times ($p < 0.05$). There were no significant differences in blood loss, postoperative drainage and postoperative CK content between the two groups ($p > 0.05$). There was no difference in VAS score and ODI index during the follow-up ($p > 0.05$). There was no significant difference in the interbody fusion rate between the two groups ($p > 0.05$). There was no significant difference in the distribution of type A screws, but the type B screw in the MIS-TLIF group was higher ($p < 0.05$). There was no difference in the incidence of complications between the two groups ($p > 0.05$). Conclusion: The postoperative quality of life score and radiological outcomes of the two types of surgery in two-level lumbar degenerative diseases was similar, and there was no significant difference in muscle injury and complications, but the operation time and intraoperative radiation exposurewere higher than in the OPEN-TLIF group, and the pedicle screws were more likely to deviate laterally out of the vertebral body. Therefore, OPEN-TLIF is recommended for patients with lumbar degenerative diseases of two segments.

Keywords: TLIF; MIS-TLIF; lumbar degenerative disease; clinical outcome

---

1. Introduction

Lumbar degenerative disease is a common disease in spinal surgery that mostly occurs in the elderly, with main clinical manifestations such as sciatica, low back pain, and cauda equina syndrome. Recently, transforaminal lumbar interbody fusion (TLIF) has become a common surgical approach for the clinical treatment of lumbar degenerative disease [1]. The advantage of TLIF is that the nerve is exposed laterally by removing part of the facet joint, and the traction of the nerve root is reduced to avoid potential nerve injury. TLIF preserves the integrity of the posterior column by reducing the removal of the spinous process. OPEN-TLIF has been a safe and effective lumbar fusion procedure [2]. A systematic review of 192 studies concluded that OPEN-TLIF has advantages over PLIF in complication rate, blood loss, and operation duration. The clinical outcome is similar,

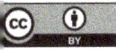

with a slightly lower postoperative ODI score for TLIF [3]. However, extensive dissection of the paraspinal muscles is required in the MIS-TLIF procedure, and this may result in postoperative paravertebral muscle atrophy and low back pain [4]

With the progress of spinal surgery technology and the development of minimally invasive surgical techniques, Foley et al. [5] proposed in 2002 to complete TLIF surgery under an expandable tube via the wistle approach, and named this minimally invasive transforaminal lumbar interbody fusion (MIS-TLIF). The decompression and fusion procedure can be operated between the multifidus muscle and longissimus muscle to reduce the injury of paraspinal muscles and soft tissues [6]. Previous studies concluded that there was no significant difference in postoperative quality of life score between Open-TLIF and MIS-TLIF [7,8], and some scholars believed that MIS-TLIF was superior to OPEN-TLIF in intraoperative blood loss and bedridden time [9,10]. However, almost all the conclusions were based on single-segment lumbar degenerative diseases [9–13], and the merits of the two surgical methods in two-segment lumbar diseases are still controversial.

With the aging of the population, patients with two segments lumbar degenerative diseases are not uncommon. According to a long-term follow-up study, about 20% of patients with lumbar degenerative diseases have two or more levels of lumbar disc herniation [14]. For these patients, multilevel surgery may be necessary, and choosing a more appropriate surgical procedure will reduce surgical trauma. Whether MIS-TLIF still has advantages for two segments degenerative lumbar diseases is still debatable. To our knowledge, there has been no literature focused on the comparison of the two surgical methods for two segments disorders. In clinical practice, we found that the two surgical methods have similar efficacy. In order to verify this hypothesis, a total of 112 patients with lumbar degenerative diseases of two segments treated in our institution from January 2015 to September 2021 were included in this study. MIS-TLIF and Open-TLIF were used for surgical treatment, and we compared the clinical and radiological outcomes of the two methods.

2. Materials and Methods

2.1. Inclusion and Exclusion Criteria

Inclusion criteria: (1) patients with typical clinical manifestations of lumbar spinal stenosis, lower extremity neurological symptoms, low back and leg pain and failed to respond to standard conservative treatment for 3 months; (2) lumbar imaging examination showed spinal stenosis with or without lumbar spondylolisthesis; (3) CT and MRI confirmed two-level disc degeneration, the abnormal changes in imaging was consistent with clinical symptoms.

Exclusion criteria: (1) deformity or combined with grade III or above lumbar spondylolisthesis; (2) lumbar infection, tumor, severe osteoporosis or motor neuron disease; (3) patients who had undergone lumbar surgery or local block therapy; (4) incomplete imaging data and loss of follow-up.

2.2. General Information of Patients

A total of 112 patients with lumbar degenerative diseases of two segments were included according to the inclusion and exclusion criteria. There were 60 patients in the OPEN-TLIF group, which was also treated as the control, including 34 males and 26 females. There were 52 patients in MIS-TLIF group, including 28 males and 24 females. There was no significant difference in preoperative general information between the two groups (Table 1). All patients were treated by experienced physicians using the Quadrant minimally invasive operating system (Beijing Fule Technology Development Co., Ltd., Beijing, China). This study was reviewed and approved by the Ethics Committee of Henan Provincial People's Hospital(IRB approval number 2021–173). All patients signed informed consent.

Table 1. General information of the two groups.

	Mis-TLIF Group (n = 52)	Open-TLIF Group (n = 60)	p Value
Age (years)	64.18 ± 8.17	66.24 ± 7.16	0.271
Gender (Male/Female)	28/24	34/26	0.322
BMI (kg/m^2)	32.41 ± 3.87	33.74 ± 4.15	0.642
Lumbar spondylolisthesis	18(18/52)	14(14/60)	0.196
Operative site			0.147
L3/4 and L4/5	16	22	
L4/5 and L5/S1	36	38	

2.3. Surgical Method of OPEN-TLIF

After general anesthesia, patients in the Open-TLIF group were placed in a prone position, and the operation area was routinely disinfected. The paravertebral muscle was separated from the spinous process, lamina, and facet capsule. The facet joints were exposed, three pedicle screws were inserted. The facet joint was bitten, the lamina was removed, the hyperplastic ligamentum flavum was removed, the dural sac and nerve roots were exposed, the protruding nucleus pulposus was removed, the intervertebral disc tissue was cleaned, the upper and lower cartilaginous endplates were scraped, the trimmed bone particles were implanted in the intervertebral space, and the cage was implanted in an oblique way. Whether to perform contralateral decompression was determined according to the preoperative symptoms and imaging manifestations. A paravertebral drainage tube was implanted, and the incision was sutured layer by layer.

2.4. Surgical Method of MIS-TLIF

The anesthesia mode and intraoperative position of patients in MIS-TLIF group were consistent with those in the OPEN-TLIF group. A posterior median incision was made, the subcutaneous skin was separated, and the skin was separated to the fascia layer on both sides. The fascia was cut 2 cm beside the midline at the intermuscular space between the longissimus muscle and multifidus muscle. A guide wire was implanted in the muscle space by blunt separation. After confirming the correct location, the quadrant channel was inserted. The remaining surgical procedures were the same as OPEN-TLIF surgery.

2.5. Postoperative Management

Prophylactic antibiotics were applied for 72 h after operation, and tower limb activity and symptom relief of patients were observed regularly. Braces were worn regularly for 3 months. Follow-up was performed at 1 week, 6 and 12 months after operation. X-ray and CT examinations were performed.

2.6. Observational Index

We used VAS score and ODI index to evaluate the clinical efficacy after the surgery. VAS score for low back pain and VAS score for leg pain and ODI index were recorded before operation, 1 week, 3 months and 12 months after operation.

Muscle injury during the perioperative period was evaluated according to the changes of blood creatine kinase (CK), and the CK content of the two groups was measured at preoperative, 3 days and 1 week after operation.

Postoperative intervertebral fusion was evaluated by the grading of lumbar fusion proposed by Bridwell et al. [15]. Grade 1 showed complete fusion of the intervertebral space with trabecular reconstruction, and the grade 2 showed incomplete fusion of the intervertebral space with trabecular reconstruction.

The screw position was evaluated by the classification proposed by Rao et al. [16]. Type A0 means that the screw did not penetrate the medial wall of the pedicle. Type A1 means that the screw penetrated the medial wall of the pedicle less than 2 mm. Type A2 means that the screw penetration of the medial wall of the pedicle was greater than 2 mm and less than 4 mm. Type B0 means that the screw did not penetrate the lateral wall of the pedicle. Type B1 means that the screw penetrated the lateral wall of the pedicle less than

2 mm. Type B2 means that the screw penetrated the lateral wall of the pedicle more than 2 mm and less than 4 mm.(Figure 1).

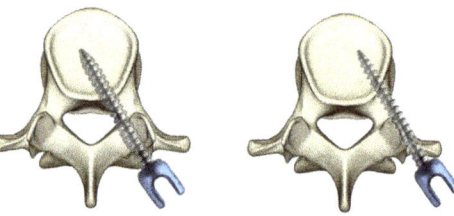

Figure 1. Diagram of type A and B screw according to RAO grading.

2.7. Statistical Analysis

SPSS 22.0(SPSS Inc., Chicago, IL, USA) was used for comparison and analysis of all data. Counting data were expressed as (X ± s). Normality of the data distribution was confirmed by Shapiro–Wilk testing. An independent sample T-test was used for comparison of the operation time, fluoroscopy, the amount of bleeding, the volume of drainage and the bed rest time between the two groups. An independent sample T-test was also used to compare the quality-of-life scores at each follow-up point between the two groups. Measurement data are expressed as (n%) and the Chi-square test was used for comparison of the general information of the patients, the complications after surgery and the distribution of screw types. Effect size (Cohen d) was calculated to examine the effect of statistical differences, and was classified as weak (≤ 0.49), moderate (0.5–0.79), or large (≥ 0.8). $p < 0.05$ was considered significant.

3. Results

3.1. Surgery Related Information

The patients were followed up for 14.7 ± 2.1 months. There were no significant differences in general information between the two groups (Table 1). Compared with the OPEN-TLIF group, the MIS-TLIF group had longer operation time, more intraoperative fluoroscopy times, but shorter postoperative bed rest time; the differences were statistically significant ($p < 0.05$). There was no significant difference in intraoperative blood loss, postoperative drainage volume ($p > 0.05$) (Table 2).

Table 2. Surgery-related indicators and complications of the two groups.

	Mis-TLIF Group (n = 52)	Open-TLIF Group (n = 60)	Cohen d	p Value
Operation time (mins)	287.74 ± 32.17	232.96 ± 42.56	1.45	0.014
Fluoroscopy	12.74 ± 2.35	7.56 ± 3.21	1.84	0.032
Amount of bleeding (mL)	537.62 ± 112.78	574.97 ± 134.26	−0.30	0.184
Volume of drainage (mL)	372.86 ± 165.41	354.91 ± 143.92	0.12	0.081
Bed rest time (days)	4.50 ± 1.08	6.24 ± 1.34	−1.43	0.037
Complications				0.792
CSF leak	6	2		
Poor wound healing	0	2		
Numbness	6	4		

3.2. CK Perioperative Content

CK content was measured between the two groups at 3 and 7 days postoperatively. In both groups we found that the CK increased in the 3 days postoperatively, but the CK reached a significant decrease in the 7 days postoperatively. When we compared the CK content between the two groups, no significant differences were found at 3 and 7 days postoperatively(Figure 2).

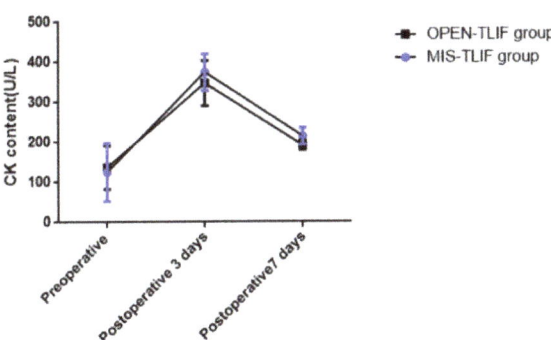

Figure 2. Changes of perioperative CK content in MIS-TLIF and Open-TLIF groups.

3.3. The Change of VAS Score and ODI Index

VAS score and ODI index was used to evaluate the clinical effect after operation. The VAS score and ODI index in the two groups were significantly improved one week after operation compared with those before operation ($p < 0.05$), and the clinical efficacy showed a trend of further improvement with the extension of follow-up time. The VAS score of low back pain in the MIS-TLIF group was lower than that in the OPEN-TLIF group 1 week after operation ($p < 0.05$), but there was no significant difference at 3 and 12 months after operation ($p > 0.05$). There was no significant difference in ODI index between the two groups at each node during follow-up ($p > 0.05$) (Tables 3–5).

Table 3. Changes in low back pain VAS score during the follow-up.

	Low Back Pain VAS Score			
	Pre-Operation	Postoperative 1 Week	Postoperative 3 Months	Postoperative 12 Months
MIS-TLIF	5.78 ± 2.12	2.03 ± 1.43 a	1.69 ± 0.72	1.19 ± 0.75
OPEN-TLIF	5.22 ± 3.37	3.11 ± 1.04	1.42 ± 0.46	1.08 ± 0.82
Cohen d	0.20	−0.86	0.45	0.14
p value	0.432	**0.012**	0.067	0.081

Table 4. Changes in leg pain VAS score during the follow-up.

	Leg Pain VAS Score			
	Pre-Operation	Postoperative 1 Week	Postoperative 3 Months	Postoperative 12 Months
MIS-TLIF	7.35 ± 1.15	2.46 ± 0.75	1.34 ± 0.87	1.04 ± 0.59
OPEN-TLIF	8.04 ± 2.01	2.45 ± 1.25	1.67 ± 0.43	1.15 ± 0.64
Cohen d	−0.42	0.01	−0.48	−0.18
p value	0.134	0.237	0.073	0.126

Table 5. Changes in ODI index during the follow-up.

	ODI (%)			
	Pre-Operation	Postoperative 1 Week	Postoperative 3 Months	Postoperative 12 Months
MIS-TLIF	76.17 ± 6.63	13.71 ± 2.38	12.26 ± 3.54	12.46 ± 4.31
OPEN-TLIF	68.42 ± 7.47	16.24 ± 3.12	15.17 ± 2.46	14.14 ± 3.37
Cohen d	1.11	−0.91	−0.95	−0.43
p value	0.243	0.176	0.102	0.065

3.4. The Screws Classified by Rao Grading

A total of 672 pedicle screws were inserted in the two groups. In the MIS-TLIF group, 360 screws were implanted, including 302 A0 screws, 46 A1 screws and 12 A2 screws. There were 214 B0 screws, 82 B1 screws and 64 B2 screws. In the OPEN-TLIF group, 312 screws were implanted, including 228 A0 screws, 54 A1 screws and 5 A2 screws. There were 242 B0 screws, 62 B1 screws and 8 B2 screws. There was no significant difference in the distribution of type A screws between the two groups ($p > 0.05$). There were significant differences in the distribution of type B screws between groups. This means that screw penetration of the lateral wall of the pedicle was more likely in the MIS-TLIF group ($p < 0.05$) (Table 6.)

Table 6. Distribution of screw types of the two groups according to RAO grading.

	OPEN-TLIF Group ($n = 360$)	MIS-TLIF Group ($n = 312$)	p Value
A type screw			0.312
A0 screw	151	124	
A1 screw	23	27	
A2 screw	6	5	
B type screw			0.021
B0 screw	107	121	
B1 screw	41	31	
B2 screw	32	4	

3.5. Fusion Level by Bridwell Grading

According to the Bridwell classification, 30 cases (57.7%) of grade 1 fusion and 22 cases (42.3%) of grade 2 fusion in the MIS-TLIF group. In the OPEN-TLIF group, 34 cases (56.7%) had grade 1 fusion and 26 cases (43.3%) had grade 2 fusion. There was no significant difference in interbody fusion rate between the two groups ($p > 0.05$).

3.6. Complications

There were no complications such as internal fixation loosening and displacement in the two groups. There were six cases of dural tear in the MIS-TLIF group and two cases in the OPEN-TLIF group, and these patients were treated with pressure dressing of the surgical incision; the drainage was removed with a delay of 1 week after operation. There were six cases in the MIS-TLIF group, and four cases in the OPEN-TLIF group experienced numbness of lower extremities; their symptoms were relieved after symptomatic treatment. There were two cases of poor wound healing in the OPEN-TLIF group, and these patients were treated with debridement and suturing. There was no significant difference in the incidence of complications between the two groups ($p > 0.05$) (Table 2).

4. Discussion

The clinical efficacy of OPEN-TLIF were verified [17,18]. Kunder et al. [17] compared the advantages and disadvantages of PLIF and OPEN-TLIF in a meta-analysis, and the results showed that OPEN-TLIF was superior to PLIF in terms of operation time, intraoperative blood loss, and incidence of complications. MIS-TLIF adopts the paravertebral space approach to complete decompression and intervertebral bone fusion through an expandable channel, which can preserve the integrity of paravertebral muscles and posterior structures of the vertebral body [19,20]. However, the channel limits the operation space, experienced surgical techniques and necessary surgical tools are required, and the learning curve is steep [21]. In this study, we found that the postoperative quality of life score and radiological outcomes of the two methods was similar but the operation time and intraoperative radiation exposure were higher in the MIS-TLIF group. A typical case is shown in Figure 3.

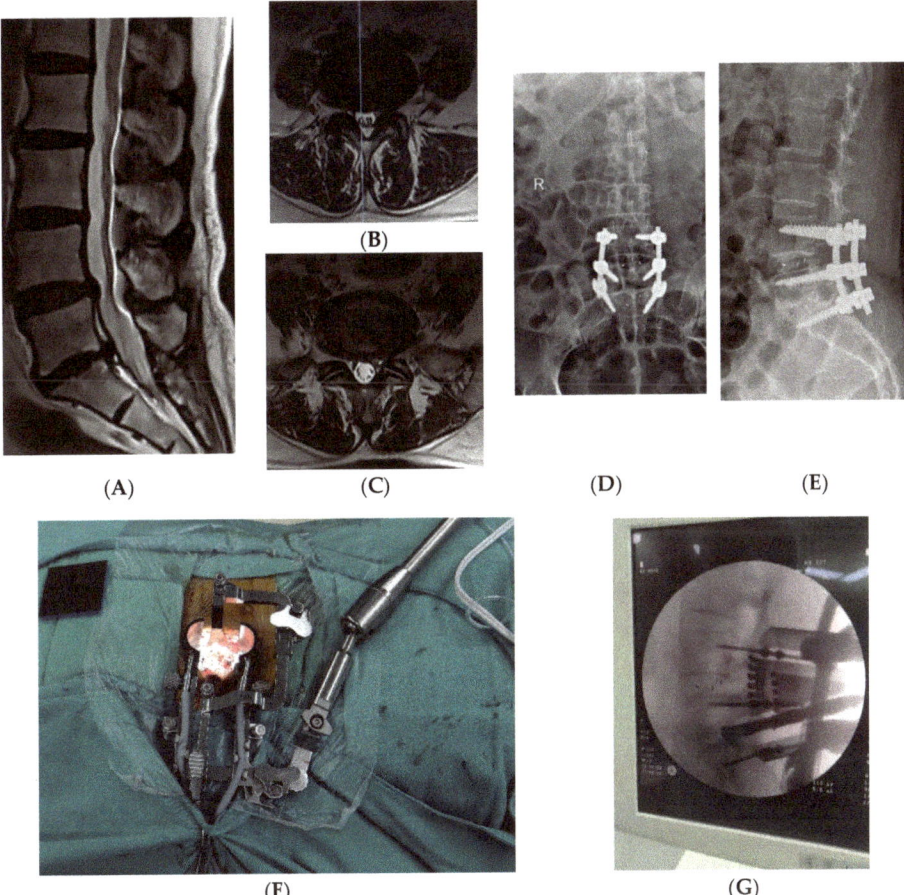

Figure 3. A typical case in the MIS-TLIF group. A 64-year-old woman was admitted to the hospital because of "waist pain for more than 10 years, aggravated with lower limb discomfort for 3 months", and underwent two-stage Mis-TLIF surgery. (**A–C**) show MRI imaging examination of disc herniation in L4/5 and L5/S1, disc degeneration in L5/S1, and narrowing of intervertebral space. (**D,E**) show postoperative X-ray. (**F,G**) The Quadrant minimally invasive operating system and an intraoperative fluoroscopic image, respectively.

During follow-up we found that the VAS score of low back pain in the MIS-TLIF group was lower than that in the OPEN-TLIF group 1 week after operation ($p < 0.05$); this was the only difference in the quality-of-life score between the two groups. The VAS score of low back pain and leg pain and ODI index had no difference in other follow-up nodes. This means that the MIS-TLIF group was superior to the OPEN-TLIF group only in early relief of low back pain, but the clinical efficacy of the two groups was similar over time. Modi and Berkman demonstrated that both techniques have the similar efficacy in single-stage lumbar degenerative disease. Our study demonstrated that the efficacy was comparable when the indications for surgery were expanded to include two-level lumbar degenerative disease [22,23].

We found that the MIS-TLIF group had higher operation time and fluoroscopy times. The increase of fluoroscopy prolonged the operation time and increased radiation exposure to doctors and patients. A number of studies have also confirmed this conclusion [24,25]. Arif et al. [26] found that the operation time of MIS-TLIF was increased by 126.3 min and fluoroscopy time was increased by 22.9 s compared with the traditional method. By monitoring the exposure dose, related research found that the radiation dose of MIS-TLIF surgery was 30 μSV higher than conventional surgery.

CK levels measured at 3 and 7 days after surgery were similar in the two groups. Muscle injury results in an increase in cell membrane passage, which leads to the release of CK into the bloodstream. Continuous monitoring of CK after surgery showed that there was no significant difference in muscle injury between the two groups. MIS-TLIF surgery is designed to minimize muscle irritation, but our study found that when MIS-TLIF was extended to 2-level surgery, the results of muscle injury did not improve compared with OPEN-TLIF.

According to Bridwell classification, there was no significant difference in the postoperative interbody fusion rate between the two groups ($p < 0.05$). This means the surgery method did not affect the fusion rate. Kang et al. [18] found that there was no significant difference in interbody fusion rate between MIS-TLIF (RR = 2.13, 95%CI: 1.39–3.27) and OPEN-TLIF (RR = 2.13, 95%CI: 1.39–3.27). This is consistent with the results of our study. Kim et al. [13] conducted a 5-year follow-up study on the fusion results of MIS-TLIF, and the authors found that the fusion rate was 97.7%. All these studies showed that the postoperative fusion rate could achieve satisfactory results whether open or minimally invasive.

In this study, we found no significant difference in the incidence of complications between the two groups. However, concerning dural tear, we found the incidence of dural tear was higher in the MIS-TLIF group. Dural tears occurred in six cases in the MIS-TLIF group and only two cases in the OPEN-TLIF group. The reason may be that the learning curve of MIS-TLIF is steep, and the operation space is narrow due to the limitation of the channel. Lee et al. [21] conducted a large sample size study to evaluate the learning curve of MIS-TLIF. The authors found that only after at least 44 cases of surgery could surgeons truly master the skill, shorten the operation time and reduce the amount of fluoroscopy, and patients could obtain satisfactory clinical efficacy. It is also worth noting that serious complications have occurred due to the surgeon's familiarity with MIS operations: duodenal rupture occurred in one case and cage loosening occurred in two cases. A study by Kang et al. [27] counted dural tears in the MIS-TLIF surgery, which occurred in one out of four patients undergoing primary surgery, and in four out of nineteen patients undergoing revision surgery. Goertz et al. [28] found that the incidence of dural tears was higher in obese patients after MIS-TLF surgery. The results of the above studies indicate that the indications for MIS-TLIF surgery should be strictly controlled, and appropriate cases should be selected to improve the safety of surgery.

In this study, there were no complications due to pedicle screw misplacement in either group. However, when the study focused on the accuracy of screw placement, and the position of the screw was evaluated according to Rao classification, the number of B-type screws in the MIS-TLIF group was higher than that in the OPEN-TLIF group ($p < 0.05$). More type B screws means that more screws broke through the lateral wall in the MIS-TLIF group. Screw penetration of the lateral wall limits screw length, reduces holding force, and may increase surgical complications. The reason may be that MIS-TLIF is performed using Quadrant channels and the narrow space may limit the angle and position of pedicle screw implantation. Previous studies have reported revision of MIS-TLIF due to postoperative neurological symptoms caused by screw misplacement. Venier et al. [29] analyzed the use of CT navigation to guide pedicle screw placement in MIS-TLIF, and the results showed that the screw placement accuracy was 95.3%, and 19 screws (4.7%) deviated into the spinal canal. The authors believed that the narrow space under the channel limited the accuracy of screw placement. The study of Zhao et al. [30] found that the injury rate of the upper facet during MIS-TLIF was 34.07% (62/182). After logistics regression analysis, the author found that a body mass index over 30 kg/m^2 and L5 pedicle screw placement were independent risk factors for facet joint injury.

This study has limitations. First, the number of cases was limited. The incidence of lumbar degenerative diseases of two segments was lower, and the lack of follow-up data for some patients further limited the sample size. Second, the follow-up time was limited. Although all the patients achieved fusion in the follow-up time of this study, the difference in long-term efficacy between the two surgical methods still needs to be observed, and the difference in long-term complications between the two surgical methods still needs to be followed up. Third, this study was a single center retrospective study. The advantages and disadvantages of the two methods should be further compared in future studies with larger sample sizes, longer follow-ups and in multiple centers.

5. Conclusions

In conclusion, the postoperative quality-of-life score and radiological outcomes of the two types of surgery in two-level lumbar degenerative diseases is similar, and there is no significant difference in muscle injury and complications. However, the operation time and intraoperative radiation exposure are higher than those of the OPEN-TLIF group, and the pedicle screws are more likely to deviate laterally out of the vertebral body. Therefore, OPEN-TLIF is recommended for patients with lumbar degenerative diseases of two segments.

Author Contributions: Conceptualization, W.H. and G.Y.; methodology, W.H.; software, H.W.; validation, W.H., K.Z. and X.W.; formal analysis, H.M.; investigation, X.W.; resources, X.W.; data curation, H.M. and K.Z.; writing—original draft preparation, W.H. and G.Y.; writing—review and editing, G.Y.; supervision, Y.G.; project administration, Y.G.; funding acquisition, Y.G. All authors have read and agreed to the published version of the manuscript.

Funding: This work was supported by the Henan Provincial Medical Science and Technology Tackling Program Joint Project (LHGJ20200047), the Henan Provincial Medical Science and Technology Tackling Program Provincial-Ministerial Co-construction Project (SB201901085), and the Henan Provincial Medical Science and Technology Tackling Program Provincial-Ministerial Co-construction Project (SBGJ2018076).

Institutional Review Board Statement: The study was conducted in accordance with the Declaration of Helsinki and approved by the Ethics Committee of Henan Provincial People's Hospital (IRB approval number 2021-173).

Informed Consent Statement: Not applicable.

Data Availability Statement: All data are described in the manuscript. The datasets used and/or analyzed in the present study are available from the corresponding author upon reasonable request.

Conflicts of Interest: The authors declare no conflict of interest.

References

1. Van Bogaert, W.; Tegner, H.; Coppieters, I.; Huysmans, E.; Nijs, J.; Moens, M.; Goudman, L.; Buyl, R.; Lundberg, M. The Predictive Value of Fear Avoidance Beliefs for Outcomes Following Surgery for Lumbar Degenerative Disease: A Systematic Review and Best Evidence Synthesis. *Pain Physician* **2022**, *25*, 441–457. [PubMed]
2. Ge, M.; Zhang, Y.; Ying, H.; Feng, C.; Li, Y.; Tian, J.; Zhao, T.; Shao, H.; Huang, Y. Comparison of hidden blood loss and clinical efficacy of percutaneous endoscopic transforaminal lumbar interbody fusion and minimally invasive transforaminal lumbar interbody fusion. *Int. Orthop.* **2022**, *46*, 2063–2070. [CrossRef] [PubMed]
3. Caelers, I.J.M.H.; de Kunder, S.L.; Rijkers, K.; van Hemert, W.L.W.; de Bie, R.A.; Evers, S.M.A.A.; van Santbrink, H. Comparison of (Partial) economic evaluations of transforaminal lumbar interbody fusion (TLIF) versus Posterior lumbar interbody fusion (PLIF) in adults with lumbar spondylolisthesis: A systematic review. *PLoS ONE* **2021**, *16*, e0245963. [CrossRef] [PubMed]
4. Putzier, M.; Hartwig, T.; Hoff, E.K.; Streitparth, F.; Strube, P. Minimally invasive TLIF leads to increased muscle sparing of the multifidus muscle but not the longissimus muscle compared with conventional PLIF-a prospective randomized clinical trial. *Spine J.* **2016**, *16*, 811–819. [CrossRef]
5. Foley, K.T.; Holly, L.T.; Schwender, J.D. Minimally invasive lumbar fusion. *Spine* **2003**, *28*, S26–S35. [CrossRef] [PubMed]
6. Leonova, O.N.; Cherepanov, E.A.; Krutko, A.V. MIS-TLIF versus O-TLIF for single-level degenerative stenosis: Study protocol for randomised controlled trial. *BMJ Open* **2021**, *11*, e041134. [CrossRef] [PubMed]
7. Lv, Y.; Chen, J.; Chen, J.; Wu, Y.; Chen, X.; Liu, Y.; Chu, Z.; Sheng, L.; Qin, R.; Chen, M. Three-year postoperative outcomes between MIS and conventional TLIF in1-segment lumbar disc herniation. *Minim Invasive Allied Technol.* **2017**, *26*, 168–176. [CrossRef] [PubMed]

8. Qin, R.; Wu, T.; Liu, H.; Zhou, B.; Zhou, P.; Zhang, X. Minimally invasive versus traditional open transforaminal lumbar interbody fusion for the treatment of low-grade degenerative spondylolisthesis: A retrospective study. *Sci. Rep.* **2020**, *10*, 21851. [CrossRef]
9. Tan, J.H.; Liu, G.; Ng, R.; Kumar, N.; Wong, H.K.; Liu, G. Is MIS-TLIF superior to open TLIF in obese patients?: A systematic review and meta-analysis. *Eur. Spine J.* **2018**, *27*, 1877–1886. [CrossRef] [PubMed]
10. Xie, L.; Wu, W.J.; Liang, Y. Comparison between Minimally Invasive Transforaminal Lumbar Interbody Fusion and Conventional Open Transforaminal Lumbar Interbody Fusion: An Updated Meta-analysis. *Chin. Med. J.* **2016**, *129*, 1969–1986. [CrossRef]
11. Droeghaag, R.; Hermans, S.M.M.; Caelers, I.J.M.H.; Evers, S.M.A.A.; van Hemert, W.L.W.; van Santbrink, H. Cost-effectiveness of open transforaminal lumbar interbody fusion (OTLIF) versus minimally invasive transforaminal lumbar interbody fusion (MITLIF): A systematic review and meta-analysis. *Spine J.* **2021**, *21*, 945–954. [CrossRef]
12. Jenkins, N.W.; Parrish, J.M.; Cha, E.D.K.; Lynch, C.P.; Sayari, A.J.; Geoghegan, C.E.; Jadczak, C.N.; Mohan, S.; Singh, K. Validation of PROMIS Physical Function in MIS TLIF: 2-Year Follow-up. *Spine* **2020**, *45*, E1516–E1522. [CrossRef] [PubMed]
13. Kim, J.S.; Jung, B.; Lee, S.H. Instrumented Minimally Invasive Spinal-Transforaminal Lumbar Interbody Fusion (MIS-TLIF): Minimum 5-Year Follow-Up With Clinical and Radiologic Outcomes. *Clin. Spine Surg.* **2018**, *31*, E302–E309. [CrossRef] [PubMed]
14. Zhou, Z.; Ni, H.J.; Zhao, W.; Gu, G.F.; Chen, J.; Zhu, Y.J.; Feng, C.B.; Gong, H.Y.; Fan, Y.S.; He, S.S. Percutaneous Endoscopic Lumbar Discectomy via Transforaminal Approach Combined with Interlaminar Approach for L4/5 and L5/S1 Two-Level Disc Herniation. *Orthop. Surg.* **2021**, *13*, 979–988. [CrossRef] [PubMed]
15. Bridwell, K.H.; Lenke, L.G.; McEnery, K.W.; Baldus, C.; Blanke, K. Anterior fresh frozen structural allografts in the thoracic and lumbar spine. Do they work if combined with posterior fusion and instrumentation in adult patients with kyphosis or anterior column defects? *Spine* **1995**, *20*, 1410–1418. [CrossRef] [PubMed]
16. Rao, G.; Brodke, D.S.; Rondina, M.; Bacchus, K.; Dailey, A.T. Inter- and intraobserver reliability of computed tomography in assessment of thoracic pedicle screw placement. *Spine* **2003**, *28*, 2527–2530. [CrossRef] [PubMed]
17. de Kunder, S.L.; van Kuijk, S.M.J.; Rijkers, K.; Caelers, I.J.M.H.; van Hemert, W.L.W.; de Bie, R.A.; van Santbrink, H. Transforaminal lumbar interbody fusion (TLIF) versus posterior lumbar interbody fusion (PLIF) in lumbar spondylolisthesis: A systematic review and meta-analysis. *Spine J.* **2017**, *17*, 1712–1721. [CrossRef] [PubMed]
18. Kang, Y.N.; Ho, Y.W.; Chu, W.; Chou, W.S.; Cheng, S.H. Effects and Safety of Lumbar Fusion Techniques in Lumbar Spondylolisthesis: A Network Meta-Analysis of Randomized Controlled Trials. *Glob. Spine J.* **2022**, *12*, 493–502. [CrossRef] [PubMed]
19. Liu, H.; Li, J.; Sun, Y.; Wang, X.; Wang, W.; Guo, L.; Zhang, F.; Zhang, P.; Zhang, W. A Comparative Study of a New Retractor-Assisted WILTSE TLIF, MIS-TLIF, and Traditional PLIF for Treatment of Single-Level Lumbar Degenerative Diseases. *Orthop. Surg.* **2022**, *14*, 1317–1330. [CrossRef] [PubMed]
20. Ali, E.M.S.; El-Hewala, T.A.; Eladawy, A.M.; Sheta, R.A. Does minimally invasive transforaminal lumbar interbody fusion (MIS-TLIF) influence functional outcomes and spinopelvic parameters in isthmic spondylolisthesis? *J. Orthop. Surg. Res.* **2022**, *17*, 272. [CrossRef] [PubMed]
21. Lee, K.H.; Yeo, W.; Soeharno, H.; Yue, W.M. Learning curve of a complex surgical technique: Minimally invasive transforaminal lumbar interbody fusion (MIS TLIF). *J. Spinal Disord. Tech.* **2014**, *27*, E234–E240. [CrossRef] [PubMed]
22. Modi, H.N.; Shrestha, U. Comparison of Clinical Outcome and Radiologic Parameters in Open TLIF Versus MIS-TLIF in Single- or Double-Level Lumbar Surgeries. *Int. J. Spine Surg.* **2021**, *15*, 962–970. [CrossRef] [PubMed]
23. Berkman, R.A.; Wright, A.H.; Khan, I.; Sivaganesan, A. Perioperative Modifications to the Open TLIF Provide Comparable Short-term Outcomes to the MIS-TLIF. *Clin. Spine Surg.* **2022**, *35*, E202–E210. [CrossRef]
24. Chen, K.; Chen, H.; Zhang, K.; Yang, P.; Sun, J.; Mo, J.; Zhou, F.; Yang, H.; Mao, H. O-arm Navigation Combined With Microscope-assisted MIS-TLIF in the Treatment of Lumbar Degenerative Disease. *Clin. Spine Surg.* **2019**, *32*, E235–E240. [CrossRef]
25. Dusad, T.; Kundnani, V.; Dutta, S.; Patel, A.; Mehta, G.; Singh, M. Comparative Prospective Study Reporting Intraoperative Parameters, Pedicle Screw Perforation, and Radiation Exposure in Navigation-Guided versus Non-navigated Fluoroscopy-Assisted Minimal Invasive Transforaminal Lumbar Interbody Fusion. *Asian Spine J.* **2018**, *12*, 309–316. [CrossRef]
26. Arif, S.; Brady, Z.; Enchev, Y.; Peev, N.; Encheva, E. Minimising radiation exposure to the surgeon in minimally invasive spine surgeries: A systematic review of 15 studies. *Orthop. Traumatol. Surg. Res.* **2021**, *107*, 102795. [CrossRef]
27. Kang, M.S.; Park, J.Y.; Kim, K.H.; Kuh, S.U.; Chin, D.K.; Kim, K.S.; Cho, Y.E. Minimally invasive transforaminal lumbar interbody fusion with unilateral pedicle screw fixation: Comparison between primary and revision surgery. *Biomed. Res. Int.* **2014**, *2014*, 919248. [CrossRef]
28. Goertz, L.; Stavrinou, P.; Hamisch, C.; Perrech, M.; Czybulka, D.M.; Mehdiani, K.; Timmer, M.; Goldbrunner, R.; Krischek, B. Impact of Obesity on Complication Rates, Clinical Outcomes, and Quality of Life after Minimally Invasive Transforaminal Lumbar Interbody Fusion. *J. Neurol. Surg. A Cent. Eur. Neurosurg.* **2021**, *82*, 147–153. [CrossRef]
29. Venier, A.; Croci, D.; Robert, T.; Distefano, D.; Presilla, S.; Scarone, P. Use of Intraoperative Computed Tomography Improves Outcome of Minimally Invasive Transforaminal Lumbar Interbody Fusion: A Single-Center Retrospective Cohort Study. *World Neurosurg.* **2021**, *148*, e572–e580. [CrossRef]
30. Zhao, Y.; Yuan, S.; Tian, Y.; Liu, X. Risk Factors Related to Superior Facet Joint Violation During Lumbar Percutaneous Pedicle Screw Placement in Minimally Invasive Transforaminal Lumbar Interbody Fusion (MIS-TLIF). *World Neurosurg.* **2020**, *139*, e716–e723. [CrossRef]

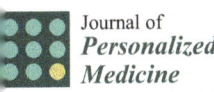

Article

Local Infiltrations in Patients with Radiculopathy or Chronic Low Back Pain Due to Segment Degeneration—Only A Diagnostic Value?

Chris Lindemann [1,*], Timo Zippelius [2], Felix Hochberger [3], Alexander Hölzl [1], Sabrina Böhle [1] and Patrick Strube [1]

1. Orthopedic Department, Jena University Hospital, Campus Eisenberg, 07607 Eisenberg, Germany
2. Department of Orthopedic Surgery, University of Ulm, 89081 Ulm, Germany
3. Department of Orthopedic Sports Medicine, Klinikum Rechts der Isar, Technical University of Munich, 81675 Munich, Germany
* Correspondence: c.lindemann@waldkliniken-eisenberg.de

Abstract: The purpose of this study was to investigate the differences in the therapeutic effectiveness of CT-assisted infiltration of a local anesthetic + corticosteroid between nerve root and facet joint capsule in patients with chronic complaints. In this prospective trial with a 12-month follow-up, a total of 250 patients with chronic low back pain and radiculopathy were assigned to two groups. In the first group, patients with specific lumbar pain due to spondyloarthritis received periarticular facet joint capsule infiltration (FJI). In the second group, patients with monoradicular pain received periradicular infiltration (PRI) via an extraforaminal selective nerve block. Clinical improvement after FJI and PRI regarding pain (NRS), function (ODI), satisfaction (McNab), and health related quality of life (SF-36) were compared. Minimally clinically important difference (MCID) served as the threshold for therapeutic effectiveness evaluation. A total of 196 patients were available for final analysis. With respect to the pain reduction and functional improvement (ODI, NRSoverall, and NRSback), the PRI group performed significantly better (ptreatment < 0.001) and longer over time (ptreatment × time 0.001) than the FJI group. Regarding pain and function, only PRI demonstrated a durable improvement larger than MCID. A significant and durable therapeutic value was found only after receiving PRI but not after FJI in patients with chronic pain.

Keywords: facet joint capsule infiltration; periradicular infiltration; selective nerve block; radiculopathy; low back pain

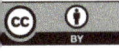

1. Introduction

Degenerative changes in the lumbar spine are a common cause of chronic pain, physical limitations, reduced health-related quality of life, and absenteeism. As a consequence, these changes are associated with considerable social and health costs in Western societies [1–5].

Facet joint degeneration, a real joint-segment-joint degeneration, is often a trigger of back pain. In addition, disc herniation, recess, or neuroforaminal stenosis often affects the nerve root and can lead to leg pain [6,7]. A variety of treatment methods are available for chronic diseases due to lumbar segment degeneration. Among these treatments, local infiltration therapy also holds differential diagnostic value.

Local anesthetics and steroids are often used here. Local anesthetics have been postulated to provide relief by various mechanisms, i.e., suppression of nociceptive discharge, the block of the sympathetic reflex arc, the blockade of the axonal transport, and anti-inflammatory effects [8]. Steroids act via two mechanisms. On one hand, steroids have anti-inflammatory, anti-edematous, and immunosuppressive properties. On the other hand, steroids inhibit neuronal transmission within C-fibers, helping to reduce both lumbar and radicular pain symptoms [6,8,9]. Furthermore, Computed Tomography (CT)-supported infiltration represents a precise and reproducible therapy option associated with reduced complication rates [10–13].

However, based on current research, the duration of the effect of therapeutically intended infiltration as it relates to the treated tissue, nerve root, or facet joint, particularly in the case of chronic and specific complaints, remains unclear. In previous studies, infiltration locations were considered partially together and partially individually compared with placebo groups, and the temporal aspect of complaint duration was insufficient [14]. However, given the different associated pathoanatomical processes (e.g., arthrosis vs. neuronal compression), differences are likely. Therefore, the aim of this study was to investigate the therapeutic value of CT-based infiltration in terms of pain, function, and quality of life based on the kind of injection (periradicular infiltration, PRI vs. facet joint capsule infiltration, FJI) in chronic complaints. We hypothesized that FJI has a shorter duration of effectiveness and therefore less therapeutic value than PRI.

2. Materials and Methods

2.1. Study Design

A total of 250 patients were screened in a single-center (university hospital, orthopedic department), prospective, nonrandomized, and nonblinded study between June 2018 and December 2019. Patients were included in the event of their consent approval. The number of cases was calculated based on the statistical parameters of the clinical outcome scores of a test cohort. The effect size for the power analysis based on a 2-sided, 2-way ANOVA with 4 or 5 measurement repetitions, and was thus set to 0.12. With a ß of 0.2 and an α of 0.05, the required group size was determined to be 86 patients. Assuming a rather conservative calculated dropout rate in telephone interviews of 45% after one year, the total group size was approximately 125 patients per group. The presented study was registered with the Trial Registry Number: DRKS00023722 (German Registry of Clinical Trials; 8 December 2020).

2.2. Ethical Approval

Study approval was obtained from the ethics committee of the University Hospital Jena, Germany (No. 5487-3/18) and all methods were performed in accordance with the relevant guidelines and regulations. All patients were informed about the study preinterventionally and gave their written informed consent to participate in the study.

2.3. Patients and Groups

The inclusion criteria were patients aged ≥ 18 years with predominantly low back pain or predominantly monoradicular leg pain after the failure of structured noninvasive conservative treatment with pain relievers and physiotherapy for at least six weeks and a complaint duration of at least 12 weeks. This includes exercise, paracetamol or Nonsteroidal Anti-inflammatory Drugs, manual therapy, acupuncture, and spinal manipulation in patients with radiculopathy. PRI was performed in patients with predominantly unilateral lumbar radiculopathy based on single-level nerve root compression (caused by a herniated disc, stenosis of the lateral recess or neuroforamen) confirmed by morphological imaging (MRI or CT). FJI was performed in patients with predominantly specific lumbar pain due to single-level lumbar segment degeneration (Fujiwara grade $\geq 3°$ spondyloarthritis with partial additional intervertebral disc degeneration, osteochondrosis, degenerative spondylolisthesis) confirmed by morphological imaging (MRI or CT) [15]. The definition for predominant pain resulted from the highest NRS value (back vs. leg). Even if this was similar in a few cases (e.g., NRS leg 6, NRS back 5), the infiltration, if MR morphologically comprehensible, was performed at the predominantly pain-inducing site. All patients were mentally and physically capable of providing consent and processing the questionnaires. During follow-up, included patients were able to receive structured conservative therapy using analgesics and physical therapy.

The exclusion criteria included previous surgeries on the affected spine segment, multilevel pathologies in the MRI of the lumbar spine, and bilateral radicular complaints. Furthermore, patients in whom the peri-interventional risk profile was increased due to other diseases were excluded. These diseases included insufficiently controlled diabetes mellitus, intake of oral anticoagulants, clotting disorders, increased laboratory infection parameters (leukocytosis and increased C-reactive protein, and known infections and/or cancer diseases. Patients who had an absolute surgical indication due to acute serious neurological deficits (e.g., paresis > 3/5 according to Janda and conus/cauda syndrome) were also excluded from the study. In addition, patients who could not meet the requirements for telephone interviews and patients with a known allergy to local anesthetics (LA) or corticosteroids were excluded from the study. Patients were consecutively assigned into two groups depending on the site of infiltration. Patients with lumbar pain due to facet joint arthrosis received FJI (FJI group), whereas patients with radicular pain due to nerve root affection received a PRI (PRI group).

2.4. Intervention

All patients were placed prone on the table for the computer tomography scanner (BrightSpeed, Manuf. GE Healthcare) and treated under sterile conditions. All interventions were standardized by a single doctor (CL). Pre-interventional oral drug sedation of the patient was performed as needed.

During FJI treatment, the needles were positioned (2× disposable cannula 1 × 120 mm, Manuf. TSK LABORATORY) after appropriate CT-based identification. As intra-articular injection is often not possible due to advanced degeneration of the facet joints, the needles were placed directly around the affected facet joint capsules (joint line, Figure 1). With regard to the inclusion criteria (single-level pathologies), only the affected facet joint pair was infiltrated. With PRI, the needles were positioned lateral to the midline at the level of the affected nerve root via an extraforaminal approach (analogous to a selective nerve root block). This prevented penetration into the epidural space, and the medication was rinsed around the affected nerve root (Figure 1). The medications used included 1.5 mL local anesthetic (1% Xylocitin®®, MIBE GmbH Arzneimittel; Lidocaine hydrochloride) + 0.5 mL corticosteroid (Lipotalon®®, Recordati Industria Chimica e Farmaceutica SpA; Dexamethasone) or only 2 mL LA in cases of steroid allergy/intolerance. No contrast agent was used in either group due to CT-secured needle positioning. Before injection, needle aspiration was performed to prevent vascular spread.

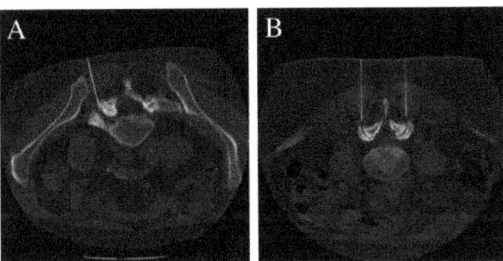

Figure 1. Computed tomography showing the positioning of the spinal needle(s) lateral to the midline at the level of the affected nerve root via an extraforaminal approach at the L5/S1 neuroforamen (**A**) and L4/5 facet joint (**B**).

2.5. Epidemiological and Clinical Data

When patients were first assessed, data, such as sex, age, weight, height, and body mass index (BMI), were recorded. In addition, grades of facet joint arthritis were determined in the FJI group using the Fujiwara classification system. In the PRI group, MR morphological differentiation of nerve root compression into moderate and advanced was performed [15].

The patient's overall pain perception was assessed using a numerical rating scale (NRSoverall 0—no pain, 10—maximum pain). Leg pain (NRSleg) and back pain (NRSback) were also assessed in isolation using the same numerical rating scale. The Oswestry Disability Index (ODI) was used to assess functional restriction [16]. The Health Short Form 36 (SF-36) was used to assess the restriction of the health-related quality of life (HrQoL) [17–19] and included evaluation of the physical (pcs) and mental (mcs) total scores. Satisfaction with the treatment was assessed using the MacNab criteria [20], with four levels of categorization: excellent, good, fair, and poor.

Pain and function (NRSoverall, NRSback, NRSleg, ODI) were assessed preprocedure and by telephone (except on day one with only NRS score) at the follow-up appointments at 6 weeks and at 3, 6, and 12 months. The SF-36 form was collected preprocedure and queried postprocedure for the 12-month follow-up.

2.6. Analysis of the Therapeutic Value

Epidemiological data and patient scores were compared between the groups. To assess the therapeutic value of PRI and FJI, the improvements in the overall pain scale and the ODI compared to the preinterventional value (deltaNRSoverall and deltaODI) were compared to the minimal clinically important difference (MCID) for chronic complaints. According to previous work, the MCID was established for pain deltaNRSoverall = 2. For function, the deltaODI = 16% [21–24].

2.7. Statistics

The statistical evaluation of this work was performed using SPSS Statistics (Version 24, IBM, Armonk, NY, USA).

The demographic data were assessed using Student's t-test for independent samples, and the normal distribution of the data was assessed in advance using the Kolmogorov–Smirnov test. Categorical data were evaluated using Fisher's exact test, and continuous data were evaluated using Student's t-test. Given that the primary and secondary target values were measured at 5 or 6 points in time, the scores were subjected to a 2-way ANOVA for repeated measures using post hoc Bonferroni tests. The Greenhouse–Geisser correction was used to assess the sphericity. A double-sided significance check was performed for all tests, and a p-value < 0.05 was assumed to indicate statistical significance for all statistical tests.

3. Results

3.1. Baseline Demographics

A total of 196 patients were available for data analysis (Figure 2). The patient baseline demographics are listed in Table 1. In the FJI group, 39 patients (45%) had infiltrated facet joints L4/5, and 48 patients (55%) had infiltrated facet joints L5/S1. In the PRI group, infiltration of the L3 nerve root occurred in 18 patients (17%), infiltration of the L4 nerve root occurred in 24 patients (22%), infiltration of the L5 nerve root occurred in 56 (51%), and infiltration of the S1 nerve root occurred in 11 patients (10%). According to the study protocol, 86 patients (99%) in the FJI group and 107 patients (98%) in the PRI group were administered an additional steroid ($p = 0.151$).

3.2. Results of Pain and Functional Improvement

All clinical scores (ODI, NRSoverall, NRSback, and NRSleg) were significantly improved over time (ptime < 0.001). With respect to the ODI, NRSoverall, and NRSback, the PRI group performed significantly better (ptreatment < 0.001) and longer over time (ptreatment × time 0.001) than the FJI group. Additionally, leg pain was significantly different between the two groups over time (ptreatment < 0.001; ptreatment × time 0.001). For detailed results and post hoc tests, see Tables 2 and 3.

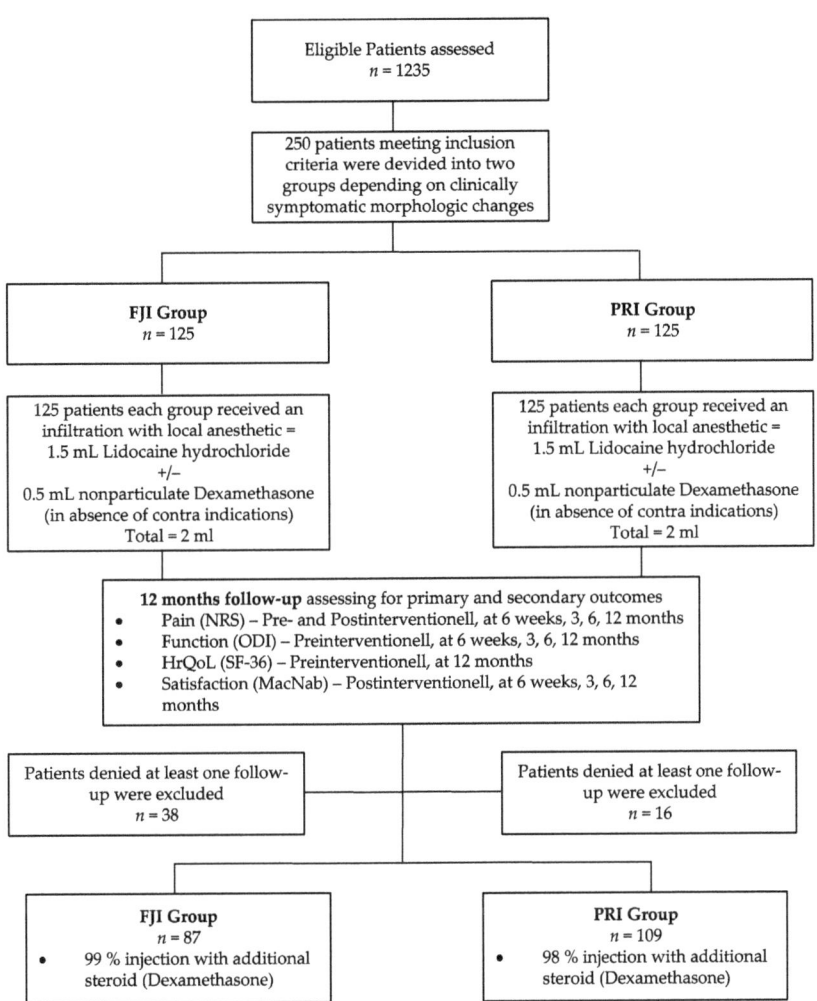

Figure 2. Flow chart. Schematic presentation of participant flow at the 12-month follow-up. FJI—facet joint capsule infiltration; PRI—periradicular infiltration therapy.

Table 1. Baseline demographic and clinical characteristics.

Groups (n = 196)		FJI Group (n = 87)	PRI Group (n = 109)	p Value
Gender	Men	38% (33)	44% (48)	0.388 *
	Woman	62% (54)	56% (61)	
Age [yrs]	Mean ± SD	66.2 ± 12.5	64.2 ± 11.6	0.248 †
Weight [kg]	Mean ± SD	83.3 ± 16.7	83.5 ± 15.9	0.935 †
Height [m]	Mean ± SD	1.7 ± 0.1	1.7 ± 0.1	0.254 †
BMI [kg/m^2]	Mean ± SD	28.8 ± 6.0	28.7 ± 5.1	0.883 †
Numeric rating scale (0–10) ‡	Mean ± SD	6.9 ± 1.2	7.1 ± 1.3	0.402 †

Table 1. Cont.

Groups (n = 196)		FJI Group (n = 87)	PRI Group (n = 109)	p Value
Oswestry Disability Index [%] (0–100)	Mean ± SD	44.4 ± 13.2	47.3 ± 17.0	0.177 [†]
Grading of facet joint arthritis (Fujiwara)	Grade 3 Grade 4			n.a.
Grading of nerve root compression	Moderate Severe	55% (48) 45% (39)	56% (61) 44% (48)	n.a.

* p-values from Fisher's exact test; [†] p-values from Student's t-test; [‡] numerical rating scale (NRS) overall including back and leg pain; SD—single standard deviation.

Table 2. Comparison of Numeric Pain Rating Scale (overall) and Oswestry Disability Index score between groups FJI and PRI over time.

Time	Numeric Pain Rating Scale		Oswestry Disability Index	
	FJI Group (87) Mean ± SD	PRI Group (109) Mean ± SD	FJI Group (87) Mean ± SD	PRI Group (109) Mean ± SD
Baseline	6.9 ± 1.2	7.1 ± 1.3	44.4 ± 13.2	47.3 ± 17.0
After intervention	1.8 * ± 1.8	1.6 * ± 1.7	-	-
6 weeks [†]	4.4 * ± 2.1	3.4 * ± 1.9	31.7 * ± 14.5	25.8 * ± 15.1
3 months [†]	5.6 * ± 1.6	3.8 * ± 2.1	37.1 * ± 11.9	26.6 * ± 14.9
6 months [†]	5.6 * ± 1.7	3.7 * ± 2.2	35.8 * ± 12.1	25.8 * ± 15.0
12 months [†]	6.2 * ± 1.8	4.4 * ± 2.5	37.8 * ± 13.4	25.6 * ± 15.1
ptreatment	<0.001		<0.001	
ptime	<0.001		<0.001	
ptreatment × time	<0.001		<0.001	

p-values from 2-sided 2-way ANOVA for repeated measures; * indicates significant improvement in posthoc tests in comparison to baseline values ($p < 0.001$); [†] indicates a significant difference in posthoc tests between the means of NRS and ODI of the 2 groups at the specified time ($p < 0.01$); ODI—Oswestry Disability Index, SD—single standard deviation.

Table 3. Comparison of Numeric Pain Rating Scale for back pain and leg pain between the groups over time.

Time	Numeric Pain Rating Scale (Back)		Numeric Pain Rating Scale (Leg)	
	FJI Group (87) Mean ± SD	PRI Group (109) Mean ± SD	FJI Group (87) Mean ± SD	PRI Group (109) Mean ± SD
Baseline [†‡]	6.9 ± 1.7	5.7 ± 1.7	4.2 ± 2.8	7.2 ± 1.7
After intervention [†]	2.4 * ± 1.6	1.3 * ± 1.4	1.2 * ± 1.7	1.8 * ± 1.4
6 weeks [†‡]	4.6 * ± 2.3	2.6 * ± 2.1	2.6 * ± 2.5	3.5 * ± 2.3
3 months [†]	5.7 * ± 1.9	2.9 * ± 2.3	3.4 * ± 2.5	3.9 * ± 2.6
6 months [†]	5.7 * ± 2.0	2.8 * ± 2.4	3.4 * ± 2.5	3.6 * ± 2.6
12 months [†]	6.0 * ± 1.9	3.6 * ± 2.6	4.5 ± 2.5	4.0 * ± 2.9
ptreatment	<0.001		0.009	
ptime	<0.001		<0.001	
ptreatment × time	<0.001		<0.001	

p-values from 2-sided 2-way ANOVA for repeated measures; * indicates significant improvement in posthoc tests in comparison to baseline values ($p < 0.001$); [†] indicates a significant difference in posthoc tests between the means of NRSback of the 2 groups at the specified time ($p < 0.05$); [‡] indicates a significant difference in posthoc tests between the means of NRSleg of the 2 groups at the specified time ($p < 0.05$) SD—single standard deviation.

3.3. Results Regarding the Therapeutic Value

Figures 3 and 4 demonstrate the improvement of pain (deltaNRSoverall) and function (deltaODI) in relation to the MCID. Here, the deltaNRSoverall failed to indicate clinical improvement in the FJI group from three months postintervention onwards, whereas the PRI group presented with clinically important improvement over the complete follow-up period. Moreover, the deltaODI of the FJI group never reached the MCID, whereas the ODI improvement of the PRI group was always greater than that of the MCID group.

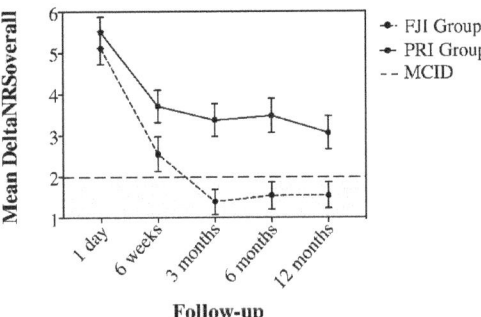

Figure 3. Comparison of deltaNRSoverall between the FJI and PRI groups over the follow-up period to illustrate the duration of the treatment effect concerning the minimal clinically important difference (MCID), (horizontal line at a DeltaNRS of 2). The FJI group fell below the horizontal line in the gray area at the 3-month follow-up, whereas the PRI group presented clinically important improvement (white area) over the complete one-year follow-up. Whiskers represent the 95% confidence interval (CI).

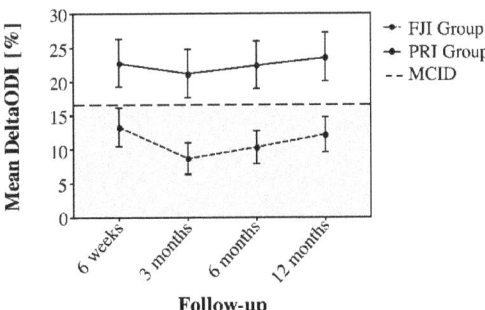

Figure 4. Comparison of deltaODI between the FJI and PRI groups over the follow-up period to illustrate the duration of the treatment effect concerning the minimal clinically important difference (MCID, horizontal line at a deltaODI of 16%). The FJI group was below the horizontal line in the gray area at the 3-month follow-up, whereas the PRI group presented clinically important improvement (white area) over the complete one-year follow-up. Whiskers represent the 95% confidence interval (CI).

3.4. Health-Related Quality of Life and Patient Satisfaction

Table 4 shows the results of the SF-36. Both groups showed similar baseline pcs values before the intervention. In contrast, patients from the FJI group showed significant deterioration in pcs ($p = 0.033$) after the intervention, whereas the PRI group showed a significant improvement in pcs ($p < 0.05$). This resulted in a significant difference in pcs between the two groups after 12 months ($p < 0.001$, Table 4).

Baseline mcs values were significantly different between the two groups ($p = 0.010$) with patients in the PRI group having a higher baseline value. Although no significant change in the baseline value was noted 12 months after the intervention in patients in the PRI group, significant deterioration in patients in the FJI group was noted ($p < 0.001$, Table 4). This resulted in worsened mcs in the FJI group at the 12-month follow-up compared to the PRI group ($p = 0.010$).

Table 4. Comparison of SF-36—physical and mental health summary scale (pcs + mcs) between the groups over time.

Time	FJI Group (87) Mean ± SD	PRI Group (109) Mean ± SD	p-Value †
SF 36 (pcs)			
Baseline	31.1 ± 6.5	32.6 ± 7.4	0.120
12 months	30.3 ± 9.4 *	35.6 ± 7.2 *	<0.001
SF 36 (mcs)			
Baseline	44.5 ± 8.3	47.8 ± 10.0	0.010
12 months	43.3 ± 9.0 *	48.3 ± 10.5	0.018

* p-values from paired samples Wilcoxon test indicates significant difference to baseline values within the group ($p < 0.05$); † p-values from Student's t-test between the groups; SD—single standard deviation.

Table 5 shows the results of patient satisfaction according to the MacNab criteria. Clear differences were noted between the groups in favor of the PRI group. A total of 92% of PRI patients (vs. 84% of FJI patients) reported excellent (complete relief of pain) or good (major relief of pain) results on the first day postintervention. Consequently, 73% (vs. 48%) of patients had excellent or good results after six weeks, 55% (vs. 27%) after three months, 53% (vs. 14%) after six months, and 51% (vs. 26%) after 12 months.

Table 5. Patients' satisfaction with infiltration therapy according to MacNab's-criteria.

Time	MacNab	FJI Group (87) Patients Treated n (%)	PRI Group (109) Patients Treated n (%)	p-Value
After intervention	Poor	3 (3)	0 (0)	
	Fair	11 (13)	9 (8)	0.007 *
	Good	42 (48)	37 (34)	
	Excellent	31 (36)	63 (58)	
6 weeks	Poor	11 (13)	2 (2)	
	Fair	34 (39)	28 (26)	<0.001 *
	Good	29 (33)	39 (36)	
	Excellent	13 (15)	40 (37)	
3 months	Poor	22 (25)	9 (8)	
	Fair	41 (47)	40 (37)	<0.001 *
	Good	12 (14)	32 (29)	
	Excellent	11 (13)	28 (26)	
6 months	Poor	35 (40)	22 (20)	
	Fair	40 (46)	29 (27)	<0.001 *
	Good	8 (9)	31 (28)	
	Excellent	4 (5)	27 (25)	
12 months	Poor	26 (30)	10 (9)	
	Fair	38 (44)	44 (40)	<0.001 *
	Good	15 (17)	28 (26)	
	Excellent	8 (9)	27 (25)	

* p-values from Fisher's exact test indicate significant difference in patients' satisfaction between the 2 groups.

3.5. Adverse Events

No differences between the groups were observed regarding the side effects after CT-based injection therapy. A total of 29 patients (15%) reported slightly transient and self-limiting side effects (1–4 h). These effects included initially increased low back pain (eight patients); numbness in the leg (ten patients); headache (seven patients); mild allergy, including redness of the face (three patients); and heartburn (one patient). Due to the self-limiting course of the side effects, no additional drug administration was necessary that could affect the outcome of the infiltration therapy. No serious adverse events were reported during the 12-month observation period.

4. Discussion

To the best of our knowledge, this study is the first to prospectively assess a direct comparison of the therapeutic value of infiltration therapies (FJI vs. PRI) in chronic complaints, under everyday clinical conditions. The study demonstrated that PRI showed a durable therapeutic effectiveness compared to FJI. Although a clinically meaningful pain reduction in back pain and possibly leg pain (MCID: NRS) was no longer detectable beyond three months after FJI, patients who received a PRI reported a clinically significant reduction in leg pain (LEP) and (if present) low back pain (LBP) over the entire period of the follow-up. The same applies to pain-associated disability in everyday life (MCID: ODI). Significant improvement in the physical health-related quality of life (SF-36: pcs) was noted in both groups, but patients who received a PRI benefited significantly more from infiltration therapy. The present results also reflect higher patient satisfaction in the PRI group.

The study demonstrates the dependence of the effectiveness of structural infiltration with local anesthetics and steroids. While a chronic neural affection seems to respond very well to the local application of the medication, arthrosis of the facet joints can only be affected to a limited extent by local therapy. The slight effect on arthritically altered joints does not seem surprising as this was also observed in other joints, such as the knee or hip joint [25,26]. The mechanism of action of a PRI with a local anesthetic and/or a steroid is probably based on neural blocking, which changes the reflex mechanism of the self-sustaining activity of the efferent fibers of the neurons and the pattern of the central neurons, thus interrupting nociceptive activity [27,28]. This pain modulation of the nerve tissue could explain the observed superior and longer-term effects of PRI despite the chronic pain characteristic of neuropathic pain. In addition, the decongestant effect of a steroid covering the affected nerve root is also observed; thus, a lower compression effect of the surrounding tissue on the nerve root is conceivable [29]. Furthermore, the natural course of both pathologies must be compared given that arthrosis typically progresses for more than a year, whereas compressed neural tissue, for example, after herniated discs, shows a clear tendency to recover even without therapeutic intervention [30,31]. Interestingly, we also found an effect of facet infiltration on leg pain and of nerve root infiltration on back pain. This controversy can be explained by accompanying muscle tone changes and functional complaints, such as sacroiliac joint disorders. Although not examined in direct comparison to the PRI, previous studies also observed a short-term pain-relieving effect of FJI in facet joint syndrome [32,33]. However, other studies examining the medium- to long-term effects of FJI on pain and function show divergent results [34–36]. The long-term relief of LBP after intra-articular steroid injections was between 18% and 63% in uncontrolled studies [37,38]. In controlled studies, the results are also inconsistent in the literature, and often no established scores were used to describe physical function [39,40]. Similar to the results of this study, Kawu et al. did not report any significant functional improvement, whereas Celik et al. indicated a significant improvement in function after six months [36,41]. However, significantly younger patients were included in the latter study, and radiologically proven facet joint arthropathy served as an exclusion criterion.

Clinically meaningful short- and long-term pain reduction after a PRI was demonstrated in other studies, which investigated the outcome of nerve root infiltration with radicular symptoms [42]. The authors reported an average pain reduction after root infiltration of 64–81% and functional improvement of 60–63%. Furthermore, Karpinnen et al. studied patients with LEP due to bony or discogenic stenosis who received a transforaminal epidural injection with an LA and steroid [39]. Analogous to the results of the present work, a significant improvement in pain (VAS) and function (ODI) was observed at the 12-month follow-up. However, no differences were noted in the placebo group, and Carette et al. found similar results regarding pain relief and functional improvement for steroid injection compared to placebo in regard to herniated discs [42]. The outcome of both studies underlines the potential of the natural course of neural convalescence with acute nerve compression, explaining the different durations of action of the FJI and PRI procedures. However, this notion must be compared to the fact that in the case of a herniated disc or spinal stenosis, infiltration of the nerve root with a local anesthetic and a steroid can prevent surgery by up to 71% (vs. 33% for the placebo group) [40]. This finding may be due to the positive effect in the acute and particularly painful phases, but only patients with chronic complaints were included in the present study. Hence, effectiveness in chronic persistent pain can be expected.

The presented study is not without limitations. First, a steroid was not applied to all patients, so the local drug composition was not completely uniform. However, the vast majority had steroid infiltrate. Based on the study design, effects attributed to the steroid versus the local anesthetic drug remain unclear. In this regard, individual studies show no major differences between local anesthetics and an LA/steroid mixture [2]. Second, because no contrast agent was used, we cannot completely exclude epidural spread, especially in the PRI group. However, the small volume applied, and the CT-guided needle position secured the selective nerve root block. However, it is not possible to determine exactly to what extent there was an allergic reaction or vascular passage in the presence of side effects. Another point is that the procedures were not compared to a placebo group. The comparison of the therapeutic effect of a PRI or FJI compared to a placebo group has already been investigated in numerous prospective studies [34,35,39,40]. However, the focus of this work was on comparing the individual PRI and FJI procedures. Therefore, a placebo group was not included.

Ultimately, there are also different infiltration techniques for the pathologies described (e.g., medial branch block vs. intraarticular infiltration vs. periarticular infiltration in patients with LBP or transforaminal vs. caudal vs. interlaminar approach in patients with LEP). Therefore, only conclusions about the techniques used can be drawn from the present study. Alternative forms of administration and application could show different durations. Thus, different effects could be observed depending on the approach used, which subsequently limits the comparability of the present work with other outcome studies that use alternative infiltration techniques.

5. Conclusions

We demonstrated that chronic back or leg pain, even when performed within a standardized setting, does not always respond equivalently to lumbar spinal needle intervention. Rather, the underlying pathology (facet joint arthritis vs. radiculopathy) seems to play a crucial role regarding therapeutic efficacy.

Based on the available results, CT-based PRI represents a suitable and easy method to provide long-acting therapy to patients with chronic radicular pain and associated LBP. Additionally, based on our study's clinical results, infiltration of facet joints holds no notably durable therapeutic value and may be used as a diagnostic tool only to secure the potential cause of the complaint. Alternative forms of therapy, such as facet joint radiofrequency denervation, surgical procedures, and multimodal concepts, should be considered in this regard.

Author Contributions: Conceptualization, C.L. and P.S.; methodology, P.S.; validation, P.S., C.L. and F.H.; formal analysis, P.S.; investigation, P.S.; resources, P.S.; data curation, F.H. and S.B.; writing—original draft preparation, C.L.; writing—review and editing, C.L.; visualization, A.H.; supervision, T.Z.; project administration, F.H. All authors have read and agreed to the published version of the manuscript.

Funding: This research received no external funding.

Institutional Review Board Statement: The study was conducted in accordance with the Declaration of Helsinki, and approved by the Institutional Review Board (or Ethics Committee) of University Hospital Jena, Germany (protocol code: 5487-3/18).

Informed Consent Statement: Informed consent was obtained from all subjects involved in the study.

Data Availability Statement: Not applicable.

Conflicts of Interest: The authors declare no conflict of interest.

References

1. Bachmann, S.; Oesch, P.; Knusel, O.; De Bie, R.; Van den Brandt, P.; Kool, J. Costs of long term disability in patients with non-specific low back pain; A randomized study. *Ann. Rheum. Dis.* **2006**, *65*, 609.
2. Manchikanti, L.; Boswell, M.V.; Singh, V.; Benyamin, R.M.; Fellows, B.; Abdi, S.; Buenaventura, R.M.; Conn, A.; Datta, S.; Derby, R.; et al. Comprehensive Evidence-Based Guidelines for Interventional Techniques in the Management of Chronic Spinal Pain. *Pain Physician* **2009**, *12*, 699–802. [CrossRef] [PubMed]
3. Martin, B.I.; Deyo, R.A.; Mirza, S.K.; Turner, J.A.; Comstock, B.A.; Hollingworth, W.; Sullivan, S.D. Expenditures and health status among adults with back and neck problems. *JAMA* **2008**, *299*, 656–664. [CrossRef]
4. Heliovaara, M.; Sievers, K.; Impivaara, O.; Maatela, J.; Knekt, P.; Makela, M.; Aromaa, A. Descriptive epidemiology and public-health aspects of low-back pain. *Ann. Med.* **1989**, *21*, 327–333. [CrossRef]
5. Lamers, L.M.; Meerding, W.J.; Severens, J.L.; Brouwer, W.B.F. The relationship between productivity and health-related quality of life: An empirical exploration in persons with low back pain. *Qual. Life Res.* **2005**, *14*, 805–813. [CrossRef]
6. Benny, B.; Azari, P. The efficacy of lumbosacral transforaminal epidural steroid injections: A comprehensive literature review. *J. Back Musculoskelet. Rehabil.* **2011**, *24*, 67–76. [CrossRef] [PubMed]
7. Falco, F.J.E.; Manchikanti, L.; Datta, S.; Sehgal, N.; Geffert, S.; Onyewu, O.; Singh, V.; Bryce, D.A.; Benyamin, R.M.; Simopoulos, T.T.; et al. An Update of the Systematic Assessment of the Diagnostic Accuracy of Lumbar Facet Joint Nerve Blocks. *Pain Physician* **2012**, *15*, E869–E907. [CrossRef]
8. Johansson, A.; Hao, J.; Sjolund, B. Local corticosteroid application blocks transmission in normal nociceptive c-fibers. *Acta Anaesthesiol. Scand.* **1990**, *34*, 335–338. [CrossRef]
9. Filippiadis, D.K.; Kelekis, A. A review of percutaneous techniques for low back pain and neuralgia: Current trends in epidural infiltrations, intervertebral disk and facet joint therapies. *Br. J. Radiol.* **2016**, *89*, 10. [CrossRef]
10. Kelekis, A.D.; Somon, T.; Yilmaz, H.; Bize, P.; Brountzos, E.N.; Lovblad, K.; Ruefenacht, D.; Martin, J.B. Interventional spine procedures. *Eur. J. Radiol.* **2005**, *55*, 362–383. [CrossRef]
11. Lee, K.S.; Lin, C.L.; Hwang, S.L.; Howng, S.L.; Wang, C.K. Transforaminal periradicular infiltration guided by CT for unilateral sciatica—an outcome study. *Clin. Imaging* **2005**, *29*, 211–214. [CrossRef] [PubMed]
12. Santiago, F.R.; Kelekis, A.; Alvarez, L.G.; Filippiadis, D.K. Interventional Procedures of the Spine. *Semin. Musculoskelet. Radiol.* **2014**, *18*, 309–317. [CrossRef] [PubMed]
13. Leonardi, M.; Pfirrmann, C.W.; Boos, N. Injection studies in spinal disorders. *Clin. Orthop. Rel. Res.* **2006**, *443*, 168–182. [CrossRef] [PubMed]
14. Fujiwara, A.; Tamai, K.; Yamato, M.; An, H.S.; Yoshida, H.; Saotome, K.; Kurihashi, A. The relationship between facet joint osteoarthritis and disc degeneration of the lumbar spine: An MRI study. *Eur. Spine J.* **1999**, *8*, 396–401. [CrossRef] [PubMed]
15. Fairbank, J.C. Why are there different versions of the Oswestry Disability Index? *J. Neurosurg. Spine* **2014**, *20*, 83–86. [CrossRef]
16. Stewart, A.L.; Greenfield, S.; Hays, R.D.; Wells, K.; Rogers, W.H.; Berry, S.D.; McGlynn, E.A.; Ware, J.E., Jr. Functional status and well-being of patients with chronic conditions. Results from the Medical Outcomes Study. *JAMA* **1989**, *262*, 907–913. [CrossRef]
17. Stewart, A.L.; Hays, R.D.; Ware, J.E., Jr. The MOS short-form general health survey. Reliability and validity in a patient population. *Med. Care* **1988**, *26*, 724–735. [CrossRef]
18. Ware, J.E., Jr.; Sherbourne, C.D. The MOS 36-item short-form health survey (SF-36). I. Conceptual framework and item selection. *Med. Care* **1992**, *30*, 473–483. [CrossRef]
19. Macnab, I. Negative disc exploration. An analysis of the causes of nerve-root involvement in sixty-eight patients. *JBJS* **1971**, *53*, 891–903. [CrossRef]
20. Hagg, O.; Fritzell, P.; Nordwall, A.; Swedish Lumbar Spine Study, G. The clinical importance of changes in outcome scores after treatment for chronic low back pain. *Eur. Spine J.* **2003**, *12*, 12–20. [CrossRef]
21. Farrar, J.T.; Young, J.P., Jr.; LaMoreaux, L.; Werth, J.L.; Poole, R.M. Clinical importance of changes in chronic pain intensity measured on an 11-point numerical pain rating scale. *Pain* **2001**, *94*, 149–158. [CrossRef]
22. Suarez-Almazor, M.E.; Kendall, C.; Johnson, J.A.; Skeith, K.; Vincent, D. Use of health status measures in patients with low back pain in clinical settings. Comparison of specific, generic and preference-based instruments. *Rheumatology* **2000**, *39*, 783–790. [CrossRef] [PubMed]
23. Taylor, S.J.; Taylor, A.E.; Foy, M.A.; Fogg, A.J. Responsiveness of common outcome measures for patients with low back pain. *Spine* **1999**, *24*, 1805–1812. [CrossRef] [PubMed]
24. Hepper, C.T.; Halvorson, J.J.; Duncan, S.T.; Gregory, A.J.; Dunn, W.R.; Spindler, K.P. The efficacy and duration of intra-articular corticosteroid injection for knee osteoarthritis: A systematic review of level I studies. *J. Am. Acad. Orthop. Surg.* **2009**, *17*, 638–646. [CrossRef]
25. McCabe, P.S.; Maricar, N.; Parkes, M.J.; Felson, D.T.; O'Neill, T.W. The efficacy of intra-articular steroids in hip osteoarthritis: A systematic review. *Osteoarthr. Cartil.* **2016**, *24*, 1509–1517. [CrossRef]

26. Dietrich, C.L.; Smith, C.E. Epidural granuloma and intracranial hypotension resulting from cervical epidural steroid injection. *Anesthesiology* **2004**, *100*, 445–447. [CrossRef]
27. Manchikanti, L. Role of neuraxial steroids in interventional pain management. *Pain Physician* **2002**, *5*, 182–199. [CrossRef]
28. Kim, N.R.; Lee, J.W.; Jun, S.R.; Lee, I.J.; Lim, S.D.; Yeom, J.S.; Koo, K.H.; Jin, W.; Kang, H.S. Effects of epidural TNF-alpha inhibitor injection: Analysis of the pathological changes in a rat model of chronic compression of the dorsal root ganglion. *Skeletal Radiol* **2012**, *41*, 539–545. [CrossRef]
29. Benoist, M. The natural history of lumbar disc herniation and radiculopathy. *Joint Bone Spine* **2002**, *69*, 155–160. [CrossRef]
30. Delgado-Lopez, P.D.; Rodriguez-Salazar, A.; Martin-Alonso, J.; Martin-Velasco, V. Lumbar disc herniation: Natural history, role of physical examination, timing of surgery, treatment options and conflicts of interests. *Neurocirugia* **2017**, *28*, 124–134. [CrossRef]
31. Ribeiro, L.H.; Furtado, R.N.; Konai, M.S.; Andreo, A.B.; Rosenfeld, A.; Natour, J. Effect of facet joint injection versus systemic steroids in low back pain: A randomized controlled trial. *Spine* **2013**, *38*, 1995–2002. [CrossRef] [PubMed]
32. Schulte, T.L.; Pietila, T.A.; Heidenreich, J.; Brock, M.; Stendel, R. Injection therapy of lumbar facet syndrome: A prospective study. *Acta Neurochir.* **2006**, *148*, 1165–1172; discussion 1172. [CrossRef] [PubMed]
33. Lilius, G.; Laasonen, E.M.; Myllynen, P.; Harilainen, A.; Gronlund, G. Lumbar facet joint syndrome. A randomised clinical trial. *J. Bone Joint Surg. Br.* **1989**, *71*, 681–684. [CrossRef] [PubMed]
34. Carette, S.; Marcoux, S.; Truchon, R.; Grondin, C.; Gagnon, J.; Allard, Y.; Latulippe, M. A controlled trial of corticosteroid injections into facet joints for chronic low back pain. *N. Engl. J. Med.* **1991**, *325*, 1002–1007. [CrossRef]
35. Kawu, A.A.; Olawepo, A.; Salami, A.O. Facet joints infiltration: A viable alternative treatment to physiotherapy in patients with low back pain due to facet joint arthropathy. *Niger J. Clin. Pract.* **2011**, *14*, 219–222. [CrossRef]
36. Cohen, S.P.; Raja, S.N. Pathogenesis, diagnosis, and treatment of lumbar zygapophysial (facet) joint pain. *Anesthesiology* **2007**, *106*, 591–614. [CrossRef]
37. Fairbank, J.C.; Park, W.M.; McCall, I.W.; O'Brien, J.P. Apophyseal injection of local anesthetic as a diagnostic aid in primary low-back pain syndromes. *Spine* **1981**, *6*, 598–605. [CrossRef]
38. Karppinen, J.; Malmivaara, A.; Kurunlahti, M.; Kyllonen, E.; Pienimaki, T.; Nieminen, P.; Ohinmaa, A.; Tervonen, O.; Vanharanta, H. Periradicular infiltration for sciatica: A randomized controlled trial. *Spine* **2001**, *26*, 1059–1067. [CrossRef]
39. Riew, K.D.; Yin, Y.; Gilula, L.; Bridwell, K.H.; Lenke, L.G.; Lauryssen, C.; Goette, K. The effect of nerve-root injections on the need for operative treatment of lumbar radicular pain. A prospective, randomized, controlled, double-blind study. *J. Bone Joint. Surg. Am.* **2000**, *82*, 1589–1593. [CrossRef]
40. Celik, B.; Er, U.; Simsek, S.; Altug, T.; Bavbek, M. Effectiveness of lumbar zygapophysial joint blockage for low back pain. *Turk. Neurosurg.* **2011**, *21*, 467–470. [CrossRef]
41. Buenaventura, R.M.; Datta, S.; Abdi, S.; Smith, H.S. Systematic review of therapeutic lumbar transforaminal epidural steroid injections. *Pain Physician* **2009**, *12*, 233–251. [CrossRef] [PubMed]
42. Carette, S.; Leclaire, R.; Marcoux, S.; Morin, F.; Blaise, G.A.; St-Pierre, A.; Truchon, R.; Parent, F.; Levesque, J.; Bergeron, V.; et al. Epidural corticosteroid injections for sciatica due to herniated nucleus pulposus. *N. Engl. J. Med.* **1997**, *336*, 1634–1640. [CrossRef] [PubMed]

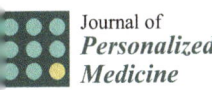

Protocol

Efficacy of Personalized Foot Orthoses in Children with Flexible Flat Foot: Protocol for a Randomized Controlled Trial

Cristina Molina-García [1], Andrés Reinoso-Cobo [2], Jonathan Cortés-Martín [3], Eva Lopezosa-Reca [2], Ana Marchena-Rodriguez [2], George Banwell [2,*] and Laura Ramos-Petersen [2]

[1] Health Sciences PhD Program, Universidad Católica de Murcia UCAM, Campus de los Jerónimos 135, 30107 Murcia, Spain; cmolina799@ucam.edu
[2] Department of Nursing and Podiatry, Faculty of Health Sciences, University of Malaga, Arquitecto Francisco Peñalosa 3, Ampliación de Campus de Teatinos, 29071 Malaga, Spain; andreicob@uma.es (A.R.-C.); evalopezosa@uma.es (E.L.-R.); amarchena@uma.es (A.M.-R.); lauraramos.94@uma.es (L.R.-P.)
[3] Research Group CTS1068, Andalusia Research Plan, Junta de Andalucia, Nursing Department, Faculty of Health Sciences, University of Granada, 18071 Granada, Spain; jcortesmartin@ugr.es
* Correspondence: gbanwell@uma.es

Abstract: Pediatric flat foot (PFF) is a very frequent entity and a common concern for parents and health professionals. There is no established definition, diagnostic method, or clear treatment approach. There are multiple conservative and surgical treatments, the implantation of foot orthoses (FO) being the most used treatment. The evidence supporting FO is very thin. It is not clearly known what the effect of these is, nor when it is convenient to recommend them. The main objective of this protocol is to design a randomized controlled trial to determine if personalized FO, together with a specific exercise regimen, produce the same or better results regarding the signs and symptoms of PFF, compared to only specific exercises. In order to respond to the stated objectives, we have proposed a randomized controlled clinical trial, in which we intend to evaluate the efficacy of FO together with strengthening exercises, compared to a control group in which placebos will be implanted as FO treatment along with the same exercises as the experimental group. For this, four measurements will be taken throughout 18 months (pre-treatment, two during treatment and finally another post-treatment measurement). The combination of FO plus exercise is expected to improve the signs and symptoms (if present) of PFF compared to exercise alone and the placebo FO group. In addition, it is expected that in both conditions the biomechanics of the foot will improve compared to the initial measurements.

Keywords: flexible flatfoot; pediatrics; children; foot orthosis; strengthening exercises

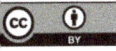

1. Introduction

Pediatric flat foot (PFF) is a very frequent syndrome in primary care consultations, and it is also a shared concern among parents and professionals. Currently, there is no clear definition for the diagnosis of PFF, no treatment protocol, nor solid scientific evidence on the wide range of treatments [1,2].

PFF is characterized by a talocalcaneal misalignment, which is reflected as a collapse of the medial longitudinal arch (MLA) in a standing position [3]. Consequently, there is excessive pronation, accompanied by a drooping of the navicular. Some feet are also accompanied by calcaneal valgus [4]. All these alterations in the morphology of the foot force the rest of the structures, such as soft tissues or joints, to compensate for the excessive forces that act on the MLA [5]. These compensations cause an inefficient gait and symptoms such as pain, fatigue, stumbling when walking, problems in the proximal joints and reduced quality of life [6,7].

Diagnosis is based on clinical findings, including a variety of clinical tests and radiographic signs, these being considered the "gold standard" [6,8,9].

Regarding treatment, there are both conservative and surgical options, surgical being the last treatment option [10]. The most common conservative treatment is the use of foot orthoses (FO), where previous studies have concluded that they improve the results of some clinical tests, radiographic angles and symptomatology [11–17]. The purpose of the FO is to modify the position of the axis of the subtalar joint, decrease the speed of pronation, support the MLA and distribute loads more effectively [18,19]. Previous systematic reviews indicate that FO are beneficial and create positive changes in the development of the child's foot [8,20,21]; these changes being greater in earlier ages of the treatment [22]. The exact age to start treatment is not clear, although it is recommended to start at preschool age (under 7 years old) so that the possibility of correcting the PFF is greater [23,24]. It has also been seen that the combination of FO with exercises is much more beneficial [25]. However, other studies indicate that the modifications that occur are those resulting from the natural development of the foot [26,27]. The evidence regarding the use of FO still does not present a consensus [20,28,29].

Therefore, there is a discrepancy between treating and not treating PFF. There are authors who conclude that it is not necessary, since the natural evolution of the foot is that the MLA begins to form at 3–4 years of age and ends at 10 years of age [26,27]. A recent meta-analysis [30] concludes that, due to the normal development of the foot, treatments should be ruled out unless there are symptoms such as pain, limited function or reduced quality of life. However, other authors recommend early treatment, based on the fact that flat feet persist in 23% of adults and may be associated with Achilles tendinopathy, plantar fasciopathy, tibial posterior tendinopathy, hallux rigidus, chondromalacia patellae or patello-femoral pain syndrome [1,2,7,13,20]. Based on these latest data, it would be unethical to leave these types of feet untreated. Additionally, a recent systematic review [24] demonstrated that FO are beneficial, with evidence regarding efficacy in treating signs and symptoms.

Therefore, since PFF is a very common syndrome which, if left untreated, could cause problems in the long term and there is no consensus on the treatment protocol, it is necessary to investigate the effectiveness of FO in terms of improvement of the signs and symptoms, including the prevention of pathologies or injuries and the improvement of the quality of life. Sagat, P et al. have shown that children with flat feet presented poor performance in certain physical tasks, in contrast to a control group with neutral feet [31]. In addition, since it is a subject of great interest for researchers, health professionals and parents, it is necessary to carry out an investigation to assess the effectiveness of FO, with a standardized diagnostic protocol with validated tests in a larger sample size than previously published studies and with a longer-term follow-up. Furthermore, as the authors Zhang J. et al. pointed out, early identification of PFF is necessary; thus an intervention plays a crucial role in enhancing the outlook. Also, there is an absence of consistent quantitative standards for diagnosing flexible flatfoot [32].

Therefore, the objective of the current study is to design a protocol for a randomized controlled trial (RCT) to determine whether personalized FO together with a specific exercise regimen produce the same or better results regarding the signs and symptoms of PFF, compared to only specific exercises. In addition, as specific objectives, to detect whether the possible bias that has prevented previous studies from demonstrating the efficacy of FO is due to the fact that these FO were not personalized; to define the PFF and to evaluate if there is a correlation between the clinical methods and the diagnosis and severity of the PFF.

2. Materials and Methods

2.1. Study Design and Setting

The design is a randomized controlled two-arm trial.

Patients will be recruited from the university clinic from Universidad Católica San Antonio de Murcia, University of Malaga and schools nearby in Spain. They will be randomized to one of the two groups, each receiving a different intervention. The schedule to follow while carrying out this RCT can be found in Appendix A. The total period intended to be allocated to this study is from September 2023 to February 2025.

To randomize the sample, a Microsoft Excel spreadsheet will be used where a random assignment sequence will be generated. Each patient will be given a consecutive number in order of arrival and allocation concealed in envelopes.

2.2. Eligibility Criteria

Subjects aged 3 to 12 years diagnosed with PFF. For the diagnosis of the PFF, the following criteria must be met:

- Foot Posture Index (FPI) > 6 [33].
- Navicular drop > 10 mm [34].
- Relaxed calcaneal stance position (RCSP) 6° to 12° valgus [35].
- Pronation angle > 10° [36].
- Arch index > a 1.35 [37].
- Double/single heel rise test negative [38].
- Windlass test negative [39].

In addition, the signature of the parents or legal guardians with consent to participate in the study will be necessary (Appendix B).

Participants will be excluded if they have undergone any surgery in the lower limbs, have previously received treatment for PFF, present osteoarticular injury, foot fractures or in the lower limbs in the last 6 months, ankle sprain, asymmetry, systemic diseases with osteoarticular involvement that present symptoms in the lower limb with gait disturbance (for example, Perthes disease) or biomechanical alteration of the lower limb with repercussions on the foot and ankle. Children suffering from any type of neurological or systemic disability (cerebral palsy, Down Syndrome, clubfoot or equino-varus, ...) will also be excluded.

2.3. Interventions

At the first visit, parents will be informed of their child's current problem, treatments, and the existence of this study. In the case of accepting to participate in the study, the process will begin: all the variables will be carefully collected, the treatment will be established and an appointment will be made for follow-up at 6 months.

First, all the affiliation data will be collected and the PFF will be diagnosed.

2.3.1. Group 1

For custom insoles, a mold will be taken using phenolic foam. To do this, the child will be asked to sit in a chair (to take the mold semi-load baring). The mold will be taken in a corrected position, that is, limiting the internal rotation of the tibia with one hand and the windlass mechanism will be performed to increase the MLA. The mold must remain neutral, so in the event that a varus or valgus print has emerged, this process will be repeated. Once we have the mold filled with plaster, two modifications will be made: a moderate medial heel skive (5 mm and an angulation of 15°) in the hindfoot and a slight inversion balance of 4° in the forefoot. Once the mold is prepared, the FO will be thermoformed; for this, we will use a 3 mm polypropylene, 25 Shore-A EVA as lining and 65 Shore-A EVA to stabilize the hindfoot.

In addition, the exercises to be performed will be explained to them and they will be given all the recommendations regarding the performance of exercises, the use of FOs and shoe therapy. These explanations will be provided in an additional report (Appendix C) that will be given to all subjects together with a calendar so that they write down all the days they perform the exercises with an X.

The exercises will first be explained by the podiatrist to the child and the parent/legal guardian. In addition, a standard video will be created so that the child can see it, in which the exercises will be explained through drawings in order to capture the attention of the child. The parent/legal guardian needs to confirm that the child is doing it correctly.

Once the FO have been provided, after assessing that it adapts well to the foot and does not cause discomfort, the patient will be requested to come in at 6 months. In the event that there is any discomfort or irritation to the child's skin, an appointment will be made to readjust or modify the FO (in this visit the variables will not be evaluated, only the FO will be fixed; if there are no problems, this visit will not be carried out).

2.3.2. Group 2

The participants will have the same intervention described for group 1, with the difference that they will use a placebo FO. This will be constructed using flat 1 mm 65 shore Ethylene-vinyl acetate (EVA), which will be cut to the foot size of the child and covered with the same top cover as the FO Group 1 to visually prevent them from being distinguished.

The instruments necessary for the development of this study and the budget necessary to carry out this clinical trial are included in Appendix D.

2.4. Outcomes Measures

The document presented in Appendix C will be used for data collection. It contains all the data to be collected in the anamnesis and all the variables to be studied, including all the clinical tests that would be carried out.

2.4.1. Qualitative or Categorical Variables:

- Gender: masculine or feminine.
- Pain: symptomatic or asymptomatic.
- Level of physical activity: high-low-nil.
- Double/simple heel rise test: Standing on toes with two legs/one leg for 25 repetitions. It will be considered positive if the participant is incapable due to fatigue or if when raising the calcaneus does not present a varus position [38].
- Supination resistance test: high-moderate-low. The patient is instructed to stand relaxed without any attempt to move the foot or lift the arch. The examiner's fingertips are then placed plantar to the medial half of the navicular, and the examiner exerts a significant lifting force on the navicular. A normal foot will demonstrate subtalar joint supination with minimal lifting force. A pes valgus deformity will need extreme amounts of lifting force in order to produce little, if any, subtalar joint supination motion [40].
- Subtalar joint axis: Lateralized-neutral-medialized. The center of the neck of the talus should be located and marked to see the lateralized or medialized point, or if, on the contrary, it stops at the 2nd finger, which would indicate that it is neutral [36].
- Shoe wear at heel level: medial-center-lateral.
- Maximum pronation test: Positive or negative. The patient is asked to try pronate as much as possible; it is considered positive when performing the maneuver, the calcaneus cannot pronate more than 2° [41].
- Forefoot: adduction-neutral-abduction position [36].
- Foot posture index (FPI): Normal = 0 to +5; pronated = +6 to +9; highly Pronated = +10 to +12; supinated = -1 to -4 and highly supinated = -5 to -12. The six clinical criteria assessed: 1. palpation of the talus head; 2. lateral supra and inframalleolar curvature; 3. position of the calcaneus in the frontal plane; 4. prominence of the talonavicular region; 5. congruence of the internal longitudinal arch and 6. abduction/adduction of the forefoot with respect to the rearfoot. As we observe them, the following score is given: neutral = 0; clear signs of supination = -2; clear signs of pronation = +2 [33].
- Test of windlass: Positive or negative. It will be considered positive if, when performing dorsiflexion of the hallux, there is not supination of the foot, plantarflexion of the 1st ray, increase in the MLA and internal rotation of the tibia [39].
- Beighton scale: Hypermobility or normal. Subjects are rated on a 9-point scale, considering 1 point for each hypermobile site. These 9 points are: 1-hyperextension of the elbows (more than 10°), 2-passively touch the forearm with the thumb, having

the wrist in flexion, 3-passive extension of the index finger to more than 90°, with the palm of the hand resting on the bed, 4-hyperextension of the knees (10° or more), patient in supine position and 5-flexion of the trunk forward touching the ground with the palms of the hands by bending without bending your knees. To be considered as hypermobile, it is required to have 4 points or more of the total of 9 [42].
- Podoscope: pronated-supinated-neutral [36].
- Pressure platform: maximum pressure zone, location of the center of gravity, gait progression line [43].

2.4.2. Quantitative or Numerical Variables

- Age: in months.
- Weight: in Kg.
- Height: in meters.
- Body Mass Index (BMI): Will be calculated with the formula weight (Kg) divided by height squared (meters^2). The classification of each child in low weight, normal weight, overweight or obesity will depend on the child's sex, height, weight and age [44].
- Pain: visual analog scale (from 1 to 10, 1 being minimum pain and 10 maximum pain).
- FPI: The six clinical criteria used in PFI are: 1. palpation of the talus head; 2. curvature supra and lateral inframaleolar region; 3. position of the calcaneus in the frontal plane; 4. prominence of the talonavicular region; 5. congruence of the internal longitudinal arch and 6. abduction/adduction of the forefoot with respect to the rearfoot. (Score: neutral = 0; clear signs of supination = -2; clear signs of pronation = $+2$) [33].
- RCSP: degrees of calcaneal eversion. The valgus degrees of the calcaneus are measured in bipedal support [35].
- Navicular drop: in millimeters. It measures the difference between the navicular position when the patient's foot is in a neutral position and when the patient's foot is in its normal position. It measures how many millimeters the medial tuberosity of the scaphoid has descended [34].
- Pronation angle: in degrees. To calculate the bisection of the distal third of the tibia with respect to the bisection of the calcaneus [36].
- Chippaux-Smirak index: in cm. On the footprint of the subject taken from a pedigraphy, the narrowest distance from the medial part of the foot (B) with the widest distance from the forefoot (A) must be measured. It is divided B/A [45].
- Pressure platform: percentage of load/weight on each foot and distribution of the same (anterior load, posterior load, load of the left and right foot) [43].
- Arch index: numerical scale. The patient's footprint is taken with a pedigraphy, the toe area is excluded and a longitudinal line is drawn that goes from the center of the heel to the 2nd toe. A line is then drawn perpendicular to the 1st. Two lines are drawn perpendicular to this axis to see the anterior extent of the forefoot area. The axis of the foot is divided into 3 equal parts and here 3 zones are defined: A: forefoot, B: midfoot and C: rearfoot. The arch index is calculated: B/(A + B + C) [37].
- Foot size: in cm.
- Silfverskiold test: in degrees. The degrees of dorsiflexion of the ankle (starting from a position of 90°) with extended knee and bent knee [46] will be measured.
- Navicular height: in millimeters. Measure the height of the scaphoid to the ground with the subject sitting [47].

2.5. Blinding and Monitoring

Participants and their parents/guardians will be blinded as to which group they are allocated to and will not see the other group.

An initial assessment will be made, these same measurements will be repeated 3 times throughout the duration of the study. In total we will obtain 4 measurements for statistical analysis.

The second measurement will be a month of treatment; in addition, in this visit we will assess the state of the FO and verify that the exercises are going well. We will ask about the FO, if any pain has appeared that was not there before, any blisters or reddened areas. In the event that the adaptation to the FO has not been good, we will make the necessary adjustments to the FO, such as lowering the MLA. If any subject needs their FO to be modified, they will be called by telephone after 2 weeks to see the evolution; in the event that it has not improved, it will be cited to re-evaluate the FO.

To corroborate that the execution of the exercises is good, we will ask the participant to repeat them, and in case there is an exercise that is not being performed correctly, we will explain it again.

The third assessment will be in the middle of the treatment/study period, that is, at 6 months. At this stage, all the initial measurements/assessments will be conducted again, as well as the last one at 12 months.

The estimated time for the measurement assessments is one hour for the 1st visit and 30 min for the rest of the visits.

2.6. Sample Size

The calculation of the sample size has been carried out with the data analysis program EPIDAT https://www.sergas.es/Saude-publica/EPIDAT?language=es (accessed on 4 August 2023). For the calculation, a clinical variation of 2 and a standard deviation of 1 have been considered. A statistical power of 80% and a significance level of $p < 0.05$; 95% confidence level. The minimum size would be a sample of 128 subjects (64 in each group randomly distributed). Considering that the loss rate could be 30%, the final size should be 84 subjects in each group. The total sample size should be 168 subjects.

2.7. Statistical Analysis

The description of data will be calculated using the percentages and frequencies of the qualitative variables and for the quantitative variables, the standard deviation and the mean. In addition, in case of presenting high deviations, the measures of central tendency would be calculated, as is the case of the mean, median or mode. All this will be carried out in frequency distribution tables of different categories, using SPSS (IBM SPSS Statistics: V.28, USA).

It is intended to compare the dependent variables with the independent ones. The Kolgorov–Smirnof test (the adjustment to the normal of the distribution) will be used to check the normality of the quantitative variables; in the event that they follow a normal distribution, the following techniques would be used: linear regression or Pearson correlation for the comparison of quantitative variables, chi-square (X^2) to compare qualitative variables and Student's t or ANOVA to compare qualitative with quantitative variables. In the event that they do not conform to the normal, it will be calculated according to the case; the Wilcoxon test, the Kruskal–Wallis test, and the Mann–Whitney test.

To determine that the supposed differences between control group and experimental group are not due to a random error, but to a real difference, in the bivariate analysis a hypothesis test will be carried out. The significance level of p shall be 0.05.

2.8. Ethics and Dissemination

The study has been awarded ethical approval from the committee of the Universidad Católica San Antonia de Murcia (CE032213).

3. Expected Results

Personalized FO along with a specific exercise regimen are expected to produce better results for signs and symptoms of PFF compared to specific exercises alone. In addition, it will be detected if the possible bias that has made the previous studies not demonstrate the efficacy of FO is that these FO were not personalized.

After the completion of this study, in which a large number of tests will be analyzed, the research will provide a definition of the PFF according to the common findings presented by the sample, a definition that nowadays is non-existent. Finally, we can evaluate if there is a correlation between clinical methods and the diagnosis and severity of PFF, in order to make an accurate diagnosis.

It is anticipated that the study will provide valuable evidence for improvement of the treatment of PFF, as well as for the diagnosis and management of this entity.

The main future research which is required after this protocol study is to carry out the detailed RCT described in the present manuscript. Also, qualitative research to understand the experience of patients with PFF wearing an FO is required.

3.1. Limitations

The main limitation that can be found in this RCT is the involvement and adherence to the study by parents or legal guardians and children. Another limitation that should be mentioned is not having a control group that does not undergo any treatment, as PFF can lead to problems in the biomechanics of gait and in the development of future pathologies. Also, we cannot claim that all patients will be using their orthoses the whole period of our study. This is because the study will be undertaken in Spain, where there are very high temperatures in summer. This may make it difficult for the patients to wear close-toed shoes, thus limiting the orthoses use and interfering with the adherence to the treatment. The use of FO will be monitored by phone, but we cannot be sure that they use them every day.

3.2. Strengths

This research will have several strengths, such as the random assignment to the treatment and the blinding of the evaluators, the direct applicability of the results obtained and the absence of quality information in this field. This research will clarify many aspects that are still unclear regarding PFF and its treatment. This section may be divided by subheadings. It should provide a concise and precise description of the experimental results, their interpretation, as well as the experimental conclusions that can be drawn.

Author Contributions: Conceptualization, C.M.-G., G.B. and L.R.-P.; methodology, C.M.-G., A.R.-C., J.C.-M., E.L.-R., A.M.-R., G.B. and L.R.-P.; writing—original draft preparation, C.M.-G., G.B. and L.R.-P.; writing—review and editing, C.M.-G., A.R.-C., J.C.-M., E.L.-R., A.M.-R., G.B. and L.R.-P. All authors have read and agreed to the published version of the manuscript.

Funding: This research received no external funding.

Institutional Review Board Statement: The study has been awarded ethical approval from the committee of the Universidad Católica San Antonia de Murcia (CE032213).

Informed Consent Statement: Not applicable.

Data Availability Statement: No more data is available.

Conflicts of Interest: The authors declare no conflict of interest.

Appendix A. Planned Schedule for the Study

Table A1. Planned Schedule for the Study.

Time/Activities	2023					2024			2025		
	August	September	October	November	December	Full year	January	February	March	April	
Project development and patient recruitment	X										
Data collection and initiation of processing		X									
Prospective follow-up			X	X	X	X	X	X			
Data analysis									X		
Results and conclusions									X	X	
Preparation of the document										X	

Appendix B. Informed Consent and Patient Information Model

Project Title: "EFFECTIVENESS OF PERSONALIZED PLANTAR ORTHOSES IN CHILDREN WITH FLEXIBLE FLAT FEET. A RANDOMIZED CONTROLLED TRIAL"

- I have read the Information Sheet that has been given to me.
- I have asked all the questions I considered necessary about the study.
- I have received satisfactory answers to all my questions.
- I have received enough information about the study.
- I will not receive any financial compensation.
- The decision to allow the analysis of my data is completely voluntary.
- If I decide freely and voluntarily to allow the evaluation of my data and those of my child, I will have the right not to be informed of the results of the investigation.
- The evaluation of all data (clinical, demographic and background) will never pose an additional danger to my child's health.
- The information about my personal and health data will be incorporated and processed in a computerized database complying with the guarantees established by the General Data Protection Regulation, as well as Organic Law 3/2018, of December 5, Protection of Personal Data and guarantee of digital rights.
- I understand that my child's participation is voluntary.
- I understand that all of my child's data will be treated confidentially.
- I understand that I can withdraw my child from the study:

Whenever.
Without having to give any kind of explanation.
Without this decision having any impact.

With all of the above, I agree for my child to participate in this study.
Signature:
In Murcia, of of 202
ID of the parent/legal guardian:
Child's ID:
Signature of parent/legal guardian:
Signature of Investigator:

PATIENT INFORMATION

STUDY TITLE
"EFFICACY OF PERSONALIZED PLANTAR ORTHOSES IN CHILDREN WITH FLEXIBLE FLAT FEET. A RANDOMIZED CONTROLLED TRIAL"

STUDY PROMOTER
Name: Cristina Molina García
Position: Assistant lecturer/researcher
Service: University Clinic UCAM Podiatry. at the medical center: Virgen de la Caridad Medical Center (Calle Olof Palme, 9-11, 30009 Murcia).
Sanitary Registration Number: 2990106.
Phone: +34 968280023. E-mail: ucampodologia@ucam.edu
It is important that you understand before deciding whether or not to participate in this study, why this research is necessary, everything that may involve your child's participation, what will be done with the information and also the possible benefits, inconveniences or risks that may entail. Without further ado, take the time you need to do a comprehensive reading and read all the information provided below.

REASON FOR STUDY
The main reason is to know if personalized plantar orthoses together with a regimen of specific exercises produce equal or better results regarding the signs and symptoms of PFF, compared to only specific exercises.

VOLUNTARY PARTICIPATION
You should know that your child's participation in this study is completely voluntary, so you can decide not to participate, change your decision at any time, without this having any impact on you or your child.

WITHDRAWAL FROM THE STUDY
In the event that you decide to leave the study, you may do so by allowing the data obtained up to the time of withdrawal from the study to be used, or by deleting all the data obtained from your child.

PARTICIPANTS
The study is designed so that all children from 3 to 12 years old, who have flexible infant flatfoot and also do not have any neurological disease or have undergone any surgery on the lower limbs, can participate.

DESCRIPTION OF THE INTERVENTION AND THE FOLLOW-UP
The clinical trial consists of the diagnosis of flexible flatfoot and the establishment of one of the two available treatment options at random. Your child may be treated with one type or another of plantar orthoses (some specific for flatfoot and others for all types of feet) in addition to a series of specific exercises. A review would be made at one month of treatment and another at 6 months and finally, the final review of the study, 12 months after the start of treatment.
All data related to flatfoot (type of flatfoot, valgus degrees, joint mobility, if there is pain, etc.) and its evolution will be collected.

POSSIBLE BENEFITS
We find several benefits, first of all is the diagnosis of this alteration of the foot, since there are many people who do not know that they suffer from it and that it can bring problems in the long run, so preventing these future ailments would be the first and most important benefit. In addition, your child will have 3 complete and thorough biomechanical studies, so other alterations that could be missed could be detected. All interventions are completely harmless and will provide you with information about the health of your child's feet.
The cost of treatment and biomechanical studies is zero, with the possibility, once the study period is over, to continue seeing evolution or establishment of a "more correct" treatment. Universally, the results and conclusions of the study will be beneficial in the future for all children who have flexible flat feet. If we get results that show which treatment is more effective, health professionals will not have so many uncertainties for the treatment of flat feet. This way all flexible flat feet will be treated properly, and money would be saved or unnecessary surgeries.

POSSIBLE RISKS OR DISCOMFORT
According to the current literature there is no risk when treating flatfoot with plantar orthoses and exercises. In addition, the purpose of this study is to know if plantar orthoses

are really necessary for the treatment of flatfoot, so the treatment group with plantar orthoses for all types of feet would not trigger any risk either.

The discomfort could come from the adaptation to the plantar orthosis or the exercises. Some type of dermatology alterations derived from chafing or allergy to the materials of the plantar orthoses have been described, although these are not frequent.

ACCESS AND PROTECTION OF PERSONAL DATA

All data are of a personal nature and will comply with the provisions of Organic Law 3/2018, of December 5, on the Protection of Personal Data and guarantee of digital rights. According to what is established in this legislation, you could exercise all your rights (access, modification, opposition and cancellation of data). The way to exercise this right would be to address any staff working in the clinic.

All the data handled in the study will be identified through a code, which means that only the study promoter and the collaborators will be able to relate that code with the data of their child. Therefore, your identity and that of your child will not be disclosed to any person, except for exceptions such as a medical emergency or a legal requirement.

CONTACT IN CASE OF DOUBTS

If at any time you have any questions or require more information you can contact Cristina Molina García as responsible for the study at the telephone number 968 280 023 or through the email ucampodologia@ucam.edu.

Model for revocation of informed consent:

SECTION FOR THE REVOCATION OF CONSENT

I, D./D^a with DNI representative of the participant D./D^a__

I revoke the consent to participate in the study, signed above. Dated

Signature parent/legal guardian

Investigator's signature

Appendix C. Patient Medical History and Report

Table A2. Patient Medical History and Report.

ANAMNESIS.		
Name:		Identification Code:
Name and ID father/mother/legal guardian:		
Address:		Phone:
DNI:	Email:	
Date of birth:		Age:
Weight:	Height:	BMI:
Allergies:	Background:	
Standing number:	Gender: Male/Female	
Level of physical activity:		High/Medium/Low
EXPLORATION-ASSESSMENT		
IPF	Punctuation:	Pronated/Normal/Supinate
NAVICULAR DROP		(mm)
DOUBLE HEEL RISE TEST		Positive/Negative
SINGLE HEEL RISE TEST		Positive/Negative
PAIN (VAS SCALE)	Symptomatic/Asymptomatic	Punctuation:
PRCA		(degrees)

Table A2. Cont.

WINDLASS TEST	Positive/Negative	
ARC HEIGHT INDEX	Punctuation:	
MAXIMUM PRONATION TEST	Positive/Negative	
ASA AXIS	Lateralized/Neutral/Medialized	
SUPINATION RESISTANCE TEST	High/Moderate/Low	
CHIPPAUX-SMIRAK INDEX		(cm)
BEIGHTON SCALE	Punctuation:	Hyperlax/Normal
TYPE OF FOREFOOT	Abduccido/Neutral/Adducido	
FOOTWEAR	Heel level: Medial/Center/Lateral	
PODOSCOPE	Pronate/Supine/Neutral	
PRONATION ANGLE		(degrees)
SILFVERSKIOLD TEST		(degrees)
NAVICULAR HEIGHT		(mm)
PRESSURE PLATFORM		
Maximum pressure zone:		
Center of gravity		
Gait progression line		
	Left	Right
Load/weight percentage	Ant: Post:	Ant: Post:
	Left:	Dx:

REPORT EXERCISES AND RECOMMENDATIONS

Exercises to be performed:

1. Tiptoe for 1 min.
2. Walk with the outer lateral edge of the foot for 1 min.
3. Stand on tiptoe, hold on for 2 s and go down 15 times.
4. Hold a tennis ball with your heels and stand on tiptoe without the ball falling, hold 2 s and go down. Perform 15 repetitions.
5. Take marbles or pens with your toes and try to put them in a bucket or change them for 1 min.
6. Stand on a towel or paper and crumple it with your toes, make this gesture for a minute.
7. Standing try to increase the arch of the foot making the greatest possible effort, do 15 repetitions.
8. To finish, standing with a ball under the sole of the foot make pressures at different points of the foot and perform stretching of the triceps sural with extended knee and bent knee.

All exercises will be repeated twice each.

All these exercises will not structure the deformity and do not develop compensations in other body segments. With them we are working all the intrinsic and extrinsic muscles of the foot involved in children's flatfoot. The rebalancing of this musculature will cause the stabilizing function of the foot to develop, in addition to improving its correct activation during dynamics.

Using the template:

1. During the first week, the plantar orthoses should be implanted progressively, that is, on the 1st day for two hours, on the 2nd day for 4 h and so on.

2. Plantar orthoses are for daily use whenever the child is standing or walking, that is they must be worn every day for as many hours as possible.
3. They can be washed with soap and cold water.
4. Do not put them near a heat source, such as on top of a radiator.
5. If they cause discomfort or signs of inflammation, redness or blisters appear on their skin, remove their child's plantar orthoses and contact the clinic.

Footwear:

The use of correct footwear is of great importance and is considered as one more part of the treatment of flatfoot, it is also considered as a trigger of flatfoot.

Avoid wearing shoes without any type of support type flip-flops or footwear that is totally flat, without any sole.

An ideal footwear for children should have a rigid buttress, should not be small or too large (should fit the index finger between the heel and the shoe), should also have a thick sole (never heels) and should not be very rigid. Children's shoes should carry any method of adjustment such as laces or Velcro and care must be taken that they are not made of synthetic material to allow perspiration.

Appendix D. Necessary Material and Budget

MATERIALS	COST
Pressure platform, computer, stretcher, goniometer, scissors, vacuum, polisher, podoscope, printer, SPSS package, pedigraph	€0
Consumables: folios, pens, stretcher sheets, printer ink, gloves, masks, pedigraph ink	100 €
Elaboration 168 plantar orthoses: phenolic foams, plaster, polypropylene, EVA linings, glue	1680 €
Publication of the article in open access	2000 €
Presentation at congresses	700 €
TOTAL BUDGET	4480 €

References

1. Carr, J.B.; Yang, S.; Lather, L.A. Pediatric Pes Planus: A State-of-the-Art Review. *Pediatrics* **2016**, *137*, e20151230. [CrossRef] [PubMed]
2. Bauer, K.; Mosca, V.S.; Zionts, L.E. What's New in Pediatric Flatfoot? *J. Pediatr. Orthop.* **2016**, *36*, 865–869. [CrossRef]
3. Graham, M.E. Congenital talotarsal joint displacement and pes planovalgus: Evaluation, conservative management, and surgical management. *Clin. Podiatr. Med. Surg.* **2013**, *30*, 567–581. [CrossRef] [PubMed]
4. Cody, E.A.; Williamson, E.R.; Burket, J.C.; Deland, J.T.; Ellis, S.J. Correlation of talar anatomy and subtalar joint alignment on weightbearing computed tomography with radiographic flatfoot parameters. *Foot Ankle Int.* **2016**, *37*, 874–881. [CrossRef] [PubMed]
5. Prachgosin, T.; Chong, D.Y.; Leelasamran, W.; Smithmaitrie, P.; Chatpun, S. Medial longitudinal arch biomechanics evaluation during gait in subjects with flexible flatfoot. *Acta Bioeng. Biomech.* **2015**, *17*, 121–130. [PubMed]
6. Harris, E.J.; Vanore, J.V.; Thomas, J.L.; Kravitz, S.R.; Mendelson, S.A.; Mendicino, R.W.; Silvani, S.H.; Gassen, S.C.; Clinical Practice Guideline Pediatric Flatfoot Panel of the American College of Foot and Ankle Surgeons. Diagnosis and treatment of pediatric flatfoot. *J. Foot Ankle Surg.* **2004**, *43*, 341–373. [CrossRef]
7. Kothari, A.; Dixon, P.C.; Stebbins, J.; Zavatsky, A.B.; Theologis, T. Are flexible flat feet associated with proximal joint problems in children? *Gait Posture* **2016**, *45*, 204–210. [CrossRef]
8. Bresnahan, P.J.; Juanto, M.A. Pediatric Flatfeet-A Disease Entity That Demands Greater Attention and Treatment. *Front. Pediatr.* **2020**, *8*, 19. [CrossRef]
9. Hegazy, F.A.; Aboelnasr, E.A.; Salem, Y.; Zaghloul, A.A. Validity and diagnostic accuracy of foot posture Index-6 using radiographic findings as the gold standard to determine paediatric flexible flatfoot between ages of 6–18 years: A cross-sectional study. *Musculoskelet. Sci. Pract.* **2020**, *46*, 102107. [CrossRef]
10. Halabchi, F.; Mazaheri, R.; Mirshahi, M.; Abbasian, L. Pediatric Flexible Flatfoot; Clinical Aspects and Algorithmic Approach. *Iran. J. Pediatr.* **2013**, *23*, 247–260.
11. Jafarnezhadgero, A.; Mousavi, S.H.; Madadi-Shad, M.; Hijmans, J.M. Quantifying lower limb inter-joint coordination and coordination variability after four-month wearing arch support foot orthoses in children with flexible flat feet. *Hum. Mov. Sci.* **2020**, *70*, 102593. [CrossRef] [PubMed]

2. Chen, K.-C.; Chen, Y.-C.; Yeh, C.-J.; Hsieh, C.-L.; Wang, C.-H. The effect of insoles on symptomatic flatfoot in preschool-aged children: A prospective 1-year follow-up study. *Medicine* **2019**, *98*, e17074. [CrossRef] [PubMed]
3. Choi, J.Y.; Lee, D.J.; Kim, S.J.; Suh, J.S. Does the long-term use of medial arch support insole induce the radiographic structural changes for pediatric flexible flat foot?—A prospective comparative study. *Foot Ankle Surg.* **2020**, *26*, 449–456. [CrossRef] [PubMed]
4. Hsieh, R.-L.; Peng, H.-L.; Lee, W.-C. Short-term effects of customized arch support insoles on symptomatic flexible flatfoot in children: A randomized controlled trial. *Medicine* **2018**, *97*, e10655. [CrossRef] [PubMed]
5. Jafarnezhadgero, A.; Madadi-Shad, M.; Alavi-Mehr, S.M.; Granacher, U. The long-term use of foot orthoses affects walking kinematics and kinetics of children with flexible flat feet: A randomized controlled trial. *PLoS ONE* **2018**, *13*, e0205187. [CrossRef] [PubMed]
6. Ahn, S.Y.; Bok, S.K.; Kim, B.O.; Park, I.S. The Effects of Talus Control Foot Orthoses in Children with Flexible Flatfoot. *J. Am. Podiatr. Med. Assoc.* **2017**, *107*, 46–53. [CrossRef]
7. Lee, H.-J.; Lim, K.-B.; Yoo, J.; Yoon, S.-W.; Yun, H.-J.; Jeong, T.-H. Effect of Custom-Molded Foot Orthoses on Foot Pain and Balance in Children with Symptomatic Flexible Flat Feet. *Ann. Rehabil. Med.* **2015**, *39*, 905–913. [CrossRef]
8. Kirby, K.A. Subtalar joint axis location and rotational equilibrium theory of foot function. *J. Am. Podiatr. Med. Assoc.* **2001**, *91*, 465–487. [CrossRef]
9. Ball, K.A.; Afheldt, M.J. Evolution of foot orthotics—Part 1: Coherent theory or coherent practice? *J. Manip. Physiol. Ther.* **2002**, *25*, 116–124. [CrossRef]
10. Dars, S.; Uden, H.; Banwell, H.A.; Kumar, S. The effectiveness of non-surgical intervention (Foot Orthoses) for paediatric flexible pes planus: A systematic review: Update. *PLoS ONE* **2018**, *13*, e0193060. [CrossRef]
11. Choi, J.Y.; Hong, W.H.; Suh, J.S.; Han, J.H.; Lee, D.J.; Lee, Y.J. The long-term structural effect of orthoses for pediatric flexible flat foot: A systematic review. *Foot Ankle Surg.* **2020**, *26*, 181–188. [CrossRef]
12. Xu, R.; Wang, Z.; Ren, Z.; Ma, T.; Jia, Z.; Fang, S.; Jin, H. Comparative Study of the Effects of Customized 3D printed insole and Prefabricated Insole on Plantar Pressure and Comfort in Patients with Symptomatic Flatfoot. *Med. Sci. Monit. Int. Med. J. Exp. Clin. Res.* **2019**, *25*, 3510. [CrossRef] [PubMed]
13. Lee, E.C.; Kim, M.O.; Kim, H.S.; Hong, S.E. Changes in resting calcaneal stance position angle following insole fitting in children with flexible flatfoot. *Ann. Rehabil. Med.* **2017**, *41*, 257–265. [CrossRef] [PubMed]
14. Molina-Garcia, C.; Banwell, G.; Rodriguez-Blanque, R.; Sánchez-García, J.C.; Reinoso-Cobo, A.; Cortés-Martín, J.; Ramos-Petersen, L. Efficacy of Plantar Orthoses in Paediatric Flexible Flatfoot: A Five-Year Systematic Review. *Children* **2023**, *10*, 371. [CrossRef]
15. Kim, E.-K.; Kim, J.S. The effects of short foot exercises and arch support insoles on improvement in the medial longitudinal arch and dynamic balance of flexible flatfoot patients. *J. Phys. Ther. Sci.* **2016**, *28*, 3136–3139. [CrossRef]
16. Steber, S.; Kolodziej, L. Analysis of radiographic outcomes comparing foot orthosis to extra-osseous talotarsal stabilization in the treatment of recurrent talotarsal joint dislocation. *J. Min. Inv. Orthop.* **2015**, *1*, 1–11. [CrossRef]
17. Whitford, D.; Esterman, A. A randomized controlled trial of two types of in-shoe orthoses in children with flexible excess pronation of the feet. *Foot Ankle Int.* **2007**, *28*, 715–723. [CrossRef] [PubMed]
18. Evans, A.M. The flat-footed child—To treat or not to treat: What is the clinician to do? *J. Am. Podiatr. Med. Assoc.* **2008**, *98*, 386–393. [CrossRef]
19. Jane MacKenzie, A.; Rome, K.; Evans, A.M. The Efficacy of Nonsurgical Interventions for Pediatric Flexible Flat Foot: A Critical Review. *J. Pediatr. Orthop.* **2012**, *32*, 830–834. [CrossRef]
20. Evans, A.M.; Rome, K.; Carroll, M.; Hawke, F. Foot orthoses for treating paediatric flat feet. *Cochrane Database Syst. Rev.* **2022**. [CrossRef]
21. Sagat, P.; Bartik, P.; Štefan, L.; Chatzilelekas, V. Are flat feet a disadvantage in performing unilateral and bilateral explosive power and dynamic balance tests in boys? A school-based study. *BMC Musculoskelet. Disord.* **2023**, *24*, 622. [CrossRef] [PubMed]
22. Zhang, J.; Jiang, S.; Li, Y.; Yu, Y.; Lu, X.; Li, Y. Advantes in diagnosis, prevention and treatment of flexible flatfoot in children. *Chin. J. Sch. Health* **2023**, *44*, 946–950.
23. Morrison, S.C.; Ferrari, J. Inter-rater reliability of the Foot Posture Index (FPI-6) in the assessment of the paediatric foot. *J. Foot Ankle Res.* **2009**, *2*, 26. [CrossRef] [PubMed]
24. Shrader, J.A.; Popovich, J.M.; Gracey, G.C.; Danoff, J.V. Navicular drop measurement in people with rheumatoid arthritis: Interrater and intrarater reliability. *Phys. Ther.* **2005**, *85*, 656–664. [CrossRef] [PubMed]
25. Sobel, E.; Levitz, S.; Caselli, M.; Tran, M.; Lepore, F.; Lilja, E.; Sinaie, M.; Wain, E. Reevaluation of the relaxed calcaneal stance position: Reliability and normal values in children and adults. *J. Am. Podiatr. Med. Assoc.* **1999**, *89*, 258–264. [CrossRef] [PubMed]
26. Carrere, M.T.A.; Méndez, A.Á. Biomechanics of the lower extremity. 5. Exploration of the joints of the foot. *REDUCA (Nurs. Physiother. Podiatry)* **2009**, *1*. [CrossRef]
27. Cavanagh, P.R.; Rodgers, M.M. The arc index: A useful measure from footprints. *J. Biomech.* **1987**, *20*, 547–551. [CrossRef]
28. Lunsford, B.R.; Perry, J. The standing heel-rise test for ankle plantar flexion: Criterion for normal. *Phys. Ther.* **1995**, *75*, 694–698. [CrossRef]
29. Jack, E. Naviculo-cuneiform fusion in the treatment of the flat foot. *J. Bone Jt. Surg.* **1953**, *88B*, 25. [CrossRef]
30. Payne, C.; Munteanu, S.; Miller, K. Position of the subtalar joint axis and resistance of the rearfoot to supination. *J. Am. Podiatr. Med. Assoc.* **2003**, *93*, 131–135. [CrossRef]

41. From Gheluwe, B.; Kirby, K.A.; Roosen, P.; Phillips, R.D. Reliability and accuracy of biomechanical measurements of the lower extremities. *J. Am. Podiatr. Med. Assoc.* **2002**, *92*, 317–326. [CrossRef] [PubMed]
42. Giessen LJVan der Liekens, D.; Rutgers, K.J.; Hartman, A.; Mulder, P.G.; Oranje, A.P. Validation of beighton score and prevalence of connective tissue signs in 773 Dutch children. *J. Rheumatol.* **2001**, *28*, 2726–2730.
43. Xu, C.; Wen, X.X.; Huang, L.Y.; Shang, L.; Cheng, X.X.; Yan, Y.B.; Lei, W. Normal foot loading parameters and repeatability of the Footscan® platform system. *J. Foot Ankle Res.* **2017**, *10*, 30. [CrossRef] [PubMed]
44. Cole, T.J.; Flegal, K.M.; Nicholls, D.; Jackson, A.A. Body mass index cut offs to define thinness in children and adolescents: International survey. *BMJ* **2007**, *335*, 194. [CrossRef] [PubMed]
45. Gonzalez-Martin, C.; Pita-Fernandez, S.; Seoane-Pillado, T.; Lopez-Calviño, B.; Pertega-Diaz, S.; Gil-Guillen, V. Variability between Clarke's angle and Chippaux-Smirak index for the diagnosis of flat feet. *Colomb. Médica* **2017**, *48*, 25–31. [CrossRef]
46. Molund, M.; Husebye, E.E.; Nilsen, F.; Hellesnes, J.; Berdal, G.; Hvaal, K.H. Validation of a new device for measuring isolated gastrocnemius contracture and evaluation of the reliability of the Silfverskiöld test. *Foot Ankle Int.* **2018**, *39*, 960–965. [CrossRef]
47. Vinicombe, A.; Raspovic, A.; Menz, H.B. Reliability of navicular displacement measurement as a clinical indicator of foot posture. *J. Am. Podiatr. Med. Assoc.* **2001**, *91*, 262–268. [CrossRef]

Disclaimer/Publisher's Note: The statements, opinions and data contained in all publications are solely those of the individual author(s) and contributor(s) and not of MDPI and/or the editor(s). MDPI and/or the editor(s) disclaim responsibility for any injury to people or property resulting from any ideas, methods, instructions or products referred to in the content.

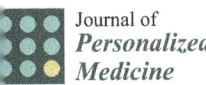

Perspective

Framing Patellar Instability: From Diagnosis to the Treatment of the First Episode

Davide Maria Maggioni [1], Riccardo Giorgino [1,2,*], Carmelo Messina [2,3], Domenico Albano [2,4], Giuseppe Michele Peretti [2,3] and Laura Mangiavini [2,3]

1. Residency Program in Orthopaedics and Traumatology, University of Milan, 20122 Milan, Italy; davidemaria.maggioni@unimi.it
2. IRCCS Istituto Ortopedico Galeazzi, 20157 Milan, Italy; carmelo.messina@unimi.it (C.M.); albanodomenico.md@gmail.com (D.A.); giuseppe.peretti@unimi.it (G.M.P.); laura.mangiavini@unimi.it (L.M.)
3. Dipartimento di Scienze Biomediche per la Salute, Università degli Studi di Milano, 20122 Milan, Italy
4. Dipartimento di Scienze Biomediche, Chirurgiche ed Odontoiatriche, Università degli Studi di Milano, Via della Commenda 10, 20122 Milan, Italy
* Correspondence: riccardo.giorgino@unimi.it; Tel.: +39-02-6621-4494

Abstract: The patellofemoral joint (PFJ) is a complex articulation between the patella and the femur which is involved in the extensor mechanism of the knee. Patellofemoral disorders can be classified into objective patellar instability, potential patellar instability, and patellofemoral pain syndrome. Anatomical factors such as trochlear dysplasia, patella alta, and the tibial tuberosity–trochlear groove (TT-TG) distance contribute to instability. Patellofemoral instability can result in various types of dislocations, and the frequency of dislocation can be categorized as recurrent, habitual, or permanent. Primary patellar dislocation requires diagnostic framing, including physical examination and imaging. Magnetic resonance imaging (MRI) is essential for assessing the extent of damage, such as bone bruises, osteochondral fractures, and medial patellofemoral ligament (MPFL) rupture. Treatment options for primary dislocation include urgent surgery for osteochondral fragments or conservative treatment for cases without lesions. Follow-up after treatment involves imaging screening and assessing principal and secondary factors of instability. Detecting and addressing these factors is crucial for preventing recurrent dislocations and optimizing patient outcomes.

Keywords: patella; instability; diagnosis; treatment; knee

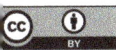

1. Introduction

The patellofemoral joint (PFJ) is a complex articulation between the patella and the femur [1,2]. The patella is the largest sesamoid of the human body. It is involved in the extensor mechanism bridging the quadriceps femoris to the proximal tibia, thus generating a transferring of forces necessary to knee extension [3].

On the other hand, the femur, with its trochlear groove, accommodates the patella. At full knee extension, the patella lays above the trochlear groove. In contrast, as the knee reaches around 30° of flexion, the patella starts engaging the trochlear groove, progressively increasing lateral translation and lateral patellar tilt [3–5]. We are therefore faced with a foul of force distribution. Anatomical structures, such as bone morphology and ligaments, in combination with adequate neuro-muscular control, play a decisive role in controlling patella–femoral kinematics [6]. Patellofemoral disorders may result.

2. Classification of Patellofemoral Disorders

The Lyonnaise school has perfected a simple and easily applicable classifying system for patellofemoral pathology by dividing it into three main groups, as follows [7]:

- *Objective patellar instability*: Patients have experienced at least one episode of patellar dislocation and present at least one or more principal factors of instability. Patellar

dislocation can occur during high-energy activities such as sports and is frequently associated with hemarthrosis.
- *Potential patellar instability*: Patients never experienced a true patellar dislocation, although they report a rather generic feeling of instability. It may occur daily during low-demand activities, such as walking and climbing stairs. These patients present one or more principal factors of instability.
- *Patellofemoral pain syndrome*: Pain is the main symptom, and it is mostly attributed to cartilage wear on either the patellar or femoral side. Imaging does not show any evident factor of instability, nor can a clinical episode of patellar dislocation be identified. In subjects suffering from patellofemoral pain (PFP) syndrome, exercise therapy should be considered the first-line treatment option as it is considered the "treatment of choice" and is supported by high-level evidence. Such therapy should include exercises for strengthening the hip and knee; these exercises can be performed through kinetic chain exercises (either weight-bearing or non-weight-bearing). Additionally, joint mobilization targeted at the knee, patellofemoral taping, and neuromuscular training have also been suggested as second-line treatment options to be used in conjunction with exercise therapy [8].

3. Principal Factors of Instability

Three main features were revealed to be relevant in knees with patellar instability that basically depend on anatomical parameters and thus on bone morphology [7]:

1. *Trochlear dysplasia* indicates whether the femoral trochlea is flat or convex (instead of concave), causing abnormal patellar tracking and a loss of joint congruence (Figures 1 and 2) Dejour classified trochlear dysplasia into four groups [9]. This classification system requires an accurate lateral X-ray (congruent posterior condyles) and confirmation via axial imaging of the knee (CT scan or MRI). A certain degree of trochlear dysplasia was found in up to 96% of patients with objective or potential patellar instability [7].
2. *Patella alta* is defined as an excessive patellar height that prevents or limits patellar engagement on the trochlea during flexion, thus predisposing the patient to patellofemoral instability. It is easily measured using the Caton–Deschamps Index (CDI) on an accurate lateral knee X-ray [10,11]. It is pathological when the CDI is greater than or equal to 1.2 (Figure 3). It is present in 30% of patellar dislocations [12].
3. *The tibial tuberosity-trochlear groove (TT-TG) distance* [13,14] is defined as the transverse length between the most prominent point of the tibial tuberosity and the trochlear groove on the femur, calculated on axial images (CT scan or MRI), representing the axial malalignment of the extensor mechanism. The greater the distance, the greater the lateralizing force acting on the patella. It is pathological when TT-TG > 13 mm on MRI or TT-TG > 20 mm on a CT scan (Figures 4 and 5).

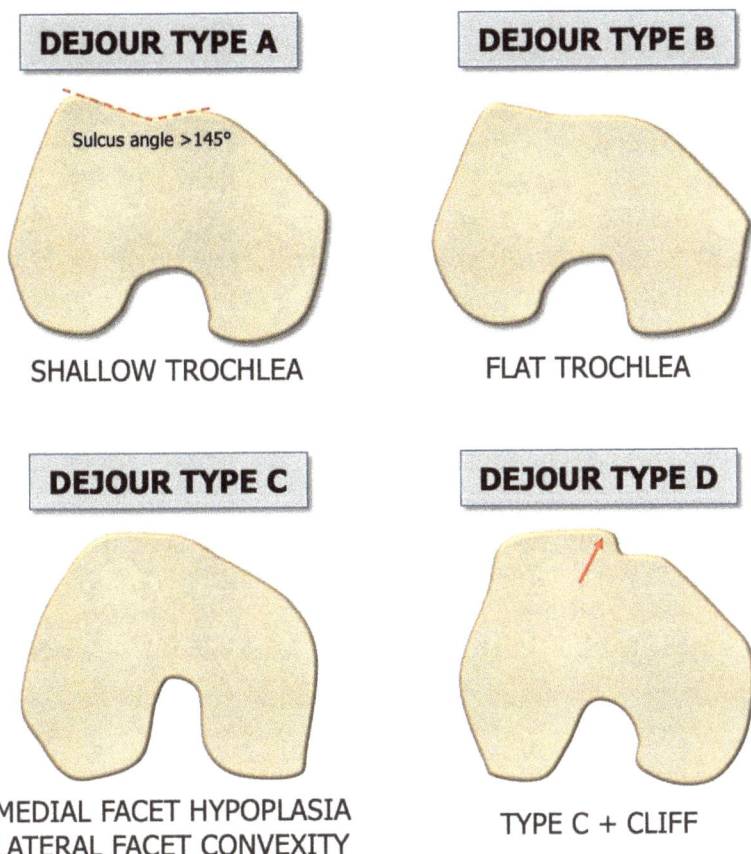

Figure 1. Dejour classification of trochlear dysplasia on axial view [7]. (Type A) Flattening of the trochlea (sulcus angle > 145°) is observed, but concavity is preserved. (Type B) The lateral facet is flat to convex with a possible supratrochlear spur. (Type C) The medial facet is hypoplastic, and the lateral facet is convex. (Type D) Complete flattening of the trochlea, with a marked depression on the medial facet (cliff sign).

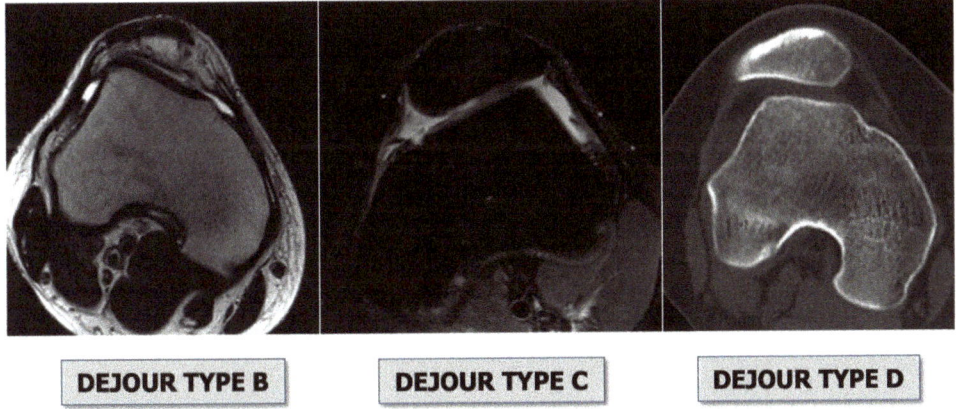

Figure 2. Types trochlear dysplasia on MRI axial view, as classified by Dejour [7].

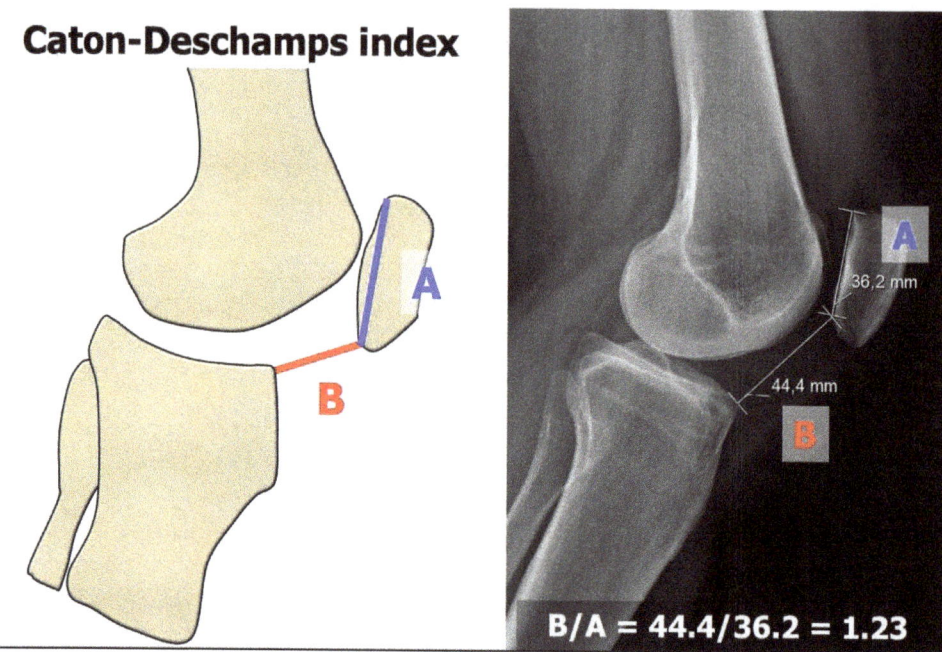

Figure 3. Caton–Deschamps Index (CDI) [10,11]. The CDI corresponds to a ratio (B/A) of the distance between the tibial plateau anterior angle to the patellar articular surface lowest aspect (B) and the patellar articular surface length (A).

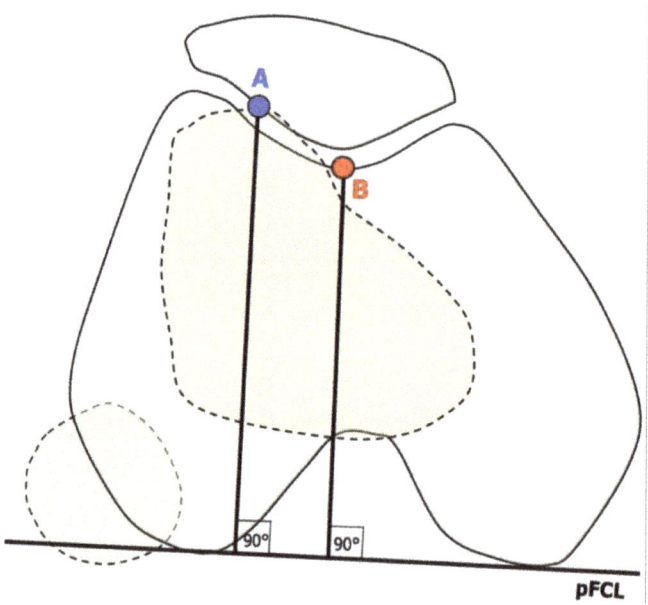

Figure 4. TT-TG distance. (A) The most prominent point of tibial tuberosity (TT). (B) Trochlear groove (TG).

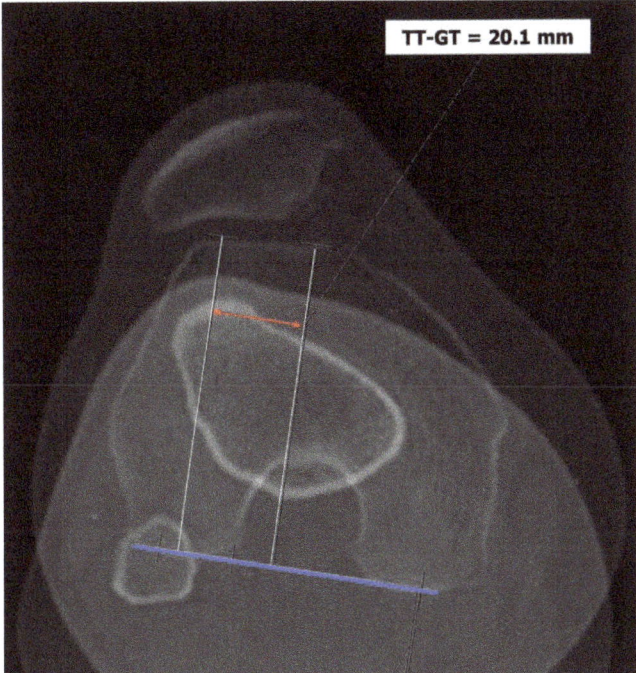

Figure 5. CT scan with pathological TT-TG of 20.1 mm.

4. Patellofemoral Instability

When patients present an anatomical predisposition (at least one principal factor of instability), the patella may incur dislocation. In general, the patella dislocates laterally as the extensor mechanism's biomechanics push toward the knee's lateral side. Other rare cases of dislocations are classified depending on the patella's position, such as medial dislocation, which is usually iatrogenic, vertical intercondylar dislocation, or horizontal intra-articular dislocation [15,16].

Patellofemoral instability can be further classified into the following categories according to the frequency of dislocation:

- Recurrent, when the patella dislocates frequently during knee flexion (two or more episodes are necessary) [17];
- Habitual, when the patella dislocates every time the knee flexes in early knee flexion (<30°) and spontaneously relocates with the extension of the knee [18].
- Permanent, when the patella is permanently dislocated through the entire knee range of motion, never facing the trochlea [19].

Dislocation is caused by a concomitance of factors, such as sports trauma, genetics, and age, to which anatomical predisposition is added.

Patellofemoral dislocation accounts for 3% of knee traumas. The average annual incidence of primary patellar dislocation has been reported to be 5.8 cases per 100,000 in the general population, with the highest incidence occurring in the second decade of life (29 per 100,000) [20]. It is more common in females and may be associated with other injuries within the knee [21]. The rate of recurrence can be up to 15–44%, and patients with a history of two or more dislocations have a 50% chance of recurrent dislocation episodes, meaning that an important slice of the population that undergoes primary patellar dislocation will not experience recurrence [22].

In 2016, Schmeling and Frosch introduced a new classification for patellar instability and maltracking, with the aim of taking into consideration both clinical and radiological pathologies [23]. This classification is based on "instability" criteria, but it also introduces the evaluation of "maltracking" criteria and "loss of patellar tracking"; overall, these factors are evaluated via both clinical and radiological aspects. Maltracking is further divided into two subtypes. According to the combination of the above factors and based on the main pathology, five types of patellar instability and maltracking are identified:

- Type 1: patellar dislocation after trauma, without instability and without patella maltracking.
- Type 2: patella instability without clinical or radiological signs of patella maltracking.
- Type 3: a combination of patella instability and patella maltracking. This type is divided into four subtypes, according to the main cause of the maltracking: (a) soft tissue contracture; (b) patella alta; (c) an abnormal tibial tuberosity–trochlea groove distance; (d) valgus deviations; and (e) torsional deformities.
- Type 4: instability and maltracking with a loss of patella tracking due to severe trochlear dysplasia, leading to a highly unstable "floating patella".
- Type 5: maltracking without instability.

This classification is advantageous because not only allows for a clear discussion of the specific case but can also be helpful in making therapy decisions as it provides surgical options for each type (and subtype).

5. Primary Dislocation: Diagnostic Framing

A patient suffering from primary patellar dislocation refers to the emergency room with a painful knee and possible flexion inability. After plain knee radiographs and an axial view of the patella, the physician performs a reduction maneuver. The patient may also arrive at the emergency room with the patella already relocated, only complaining of a painful, swollen knee. Upon physical examination, typical findings are medial side tenderness due to medial patello-femoral ligament (MPFL) rupture and a swollen knee, which may require aspiration. Patellar dislocation is a common cause of knee hemarthrosis, especially in adolescents [24].

On the X-rays, trauma surgeons must focus their attention on the following:

- Bony avulsions: depending on the size, they may require surgery [25];
- Patella alta: the CDI must be calculated. It is often the first sign of a possible PF disorder;
- Trochlear dysplasia: the crossing sign, the supra-trochlear spur, and the double contour should be identified for classification according to Dejour [9].

An MRI within a few days after the trauma is highly recommended in addition to plain radiographs [26]. Indeed, MRI allows for the detection of the following (Figures 6 and 7):

- Bone bruises on the medial side of the patella and the lateral condyle, which indicate with certainty the occurrence of a recent patellar dislocation;
- Osteochondral fracture with possible loose bodies, which are important to rule out, especially in skeletally immature patients. If the osteochondral fracture has a sufficient size (5–10 mm on MRI), urgent reduction and fixation, either open or arthroscopically, must be considered [25];
- Trochlear dysplasia, for which axial images are needed to achieve a correct classification according to the Dejour classification [9];
- MPFL rupture and location. Typically, after a patellar dislocation, the MPFL is torn [26,27]; therefore, the patella loses its major soft tissue stabilizer, which may lead to recurrent patellar instability [28].

MRI remains necessary in cases of suspected primary patellar dislocation to make a correct diagnosis, to assess concomitant osteocartilaginous injuries, and to evaluate principal factors of instability [29,30]. Recognizing the abnormalities in the bony anatomy following a primary dislocation is essential to treating patellar dislocation.

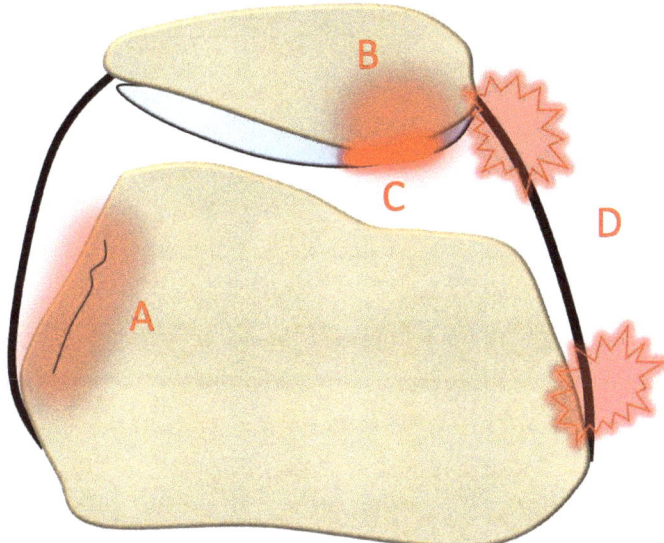

Figure 6. Consequences of acute patellar instability on the knee: (A) lateral condyle bone bruise. (B) medial patellar bone bruise. (C) patellar osteochondral damage. (D) MPFL rupture and its location, patellar insertion, mid-substance, or femoral insertion. Performing MRI within a few days from the injury is crucial to assess the patellar–femoral damages.

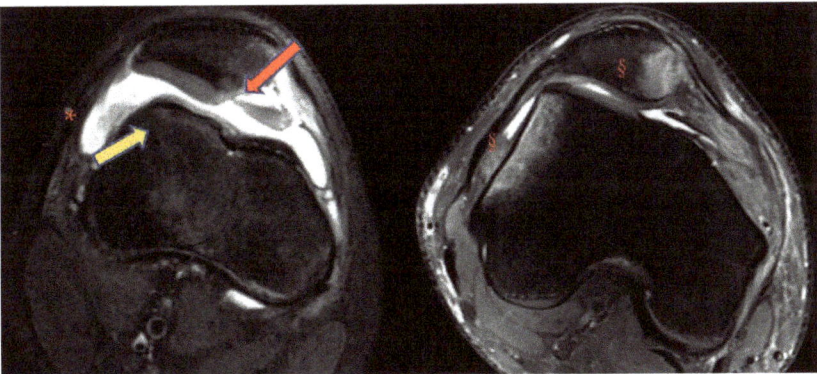

Figure 7. Case of a primary patellar dislocation, shown in MRI axial views. Note the large amount of synovial fluid or hemarthrosis (*), the bone bruise on its typical presentation (§), the chondral defect on the medial side of the patella (red arrow), and the shape of the trochlea (yellow arrow).

After the first episode, a meticulous physical examination and sufficient imaging modalities are crucial in identifying patients at a high risk of recurrence [31,32]. Skeletally immature patients are also at a higher risk of recurrence than adults. Balcarek et al. [33] proposed the "Patellar Instability Severity Score" (PISS) as a practical tool for initial risk assessment, helping to discriminate between the patients at a low risk of recurrence (PISS ≤ 3) and those at a high risk of recurrence (PISS ≥ 4, associated with a risk of recurrent dislocation up to five times greater) (Table 1). PISS is not a therapeutic algorithm; nevertheless, it may aid the orthopedic surgeon in correctly informing the patient of their condition and in being more inclined to choose a conservative or surgical approach [34]. In our opinion, it remains essential to choose an approach tailored to the patient and their condition, avoiding the so-called one-for-all approach.

Table 1. Patellar Instability Severity Score.

Age	
>16	0
≤16	1
Bilateral instability	
No	0
Yes	1
Trochlear dysplasia	
None	0
Mild (type A)	1
Severe (type B–D)	2
Patellar height, IS ratio	
≤1.2	0
>1.2	1
TT-TG distance	
<16 mm	0
≥16 mm	1
Patellar tilt	
≤20°	0
>20°	1
Total points	7

6. Primary Dislocation: Treatment Options

6.1. Urgent Surgery

Primary dislocation with a patellar osteochondral fragment is the only indication for urgent surgery [35]. The surgery consists of osteochondral fixation with pins, screws, or darts, whether absorbable or not absorbable. The dimensions of the osteochondral lesion should allow for the use of the fixation devices. MPFL reconstruction is not indicated. After surgery, an immediate rehabilitation protocol is essential. Several rehabilitation protocols exist, and they can differ according to the center and surgeon. A possible proposed protocol includes full weight bearing as the osteochondral lesion is not located in a loading zone, thereby minimizing any impact on the osteochondral fixation. Crutches are recommended for 30 days, while no brace is required. Isometric exercises for the quadriceps should be performed. Additionally, a progressive passive motion from 0° to 100° is advised for 45 days. It's important to note that the flexion of the knee can engage the patella on the trochlea, potentially affecting the osteochondral fixation. Therefore, passive motion should be stepwise to prevent any adverse effects on the fixation, though it is still necessary to avoid articular stiffness.

6.2. Conservative Treatment

In cases of dislocation without osteochondral lesions, surgery is not indicated. Arthrocentesis may relieve the patient's symptoms. Arthrocentesis also reduces the tension on the capsule and MPFL, allowing for better patellar position and decreasing pain. After surgery, an immediate rehabilitation protocol is implemented to facilitate the recovery process. This protocol includes several components:

Firstly, ice therapy is applied to help reduce swelling and manage pain in the affected area. It is typically administered intermittently for short durations. Full weight bearing is encouraged unless the osteochondral lesion is situated in a loading zone. In such cases, partial weight bearing or non-weight bearing for the first weeks may be advised to protect the affected area. Crutches are utilized for a duration of 30 days to assist with mobility and alleviate pressure on the healing joint. Light patellar bracing is employed to limit tension on the medial patellofemoral ligament (MPFL), supporting its healing and stability during the initial stages of rehabilitation. Isometric exercises of the quadriceps are prescribed to maintain muscle strength and promote stability around the knee joint. Finally, progressive passive motion exercises ranging from 0° to 100° of flexion are performed over a period of 45 days. This gradual increase in motion helps prevent joint stiffness and improve the range of motion, ensuring optimal recovery. Overall, this comprehensive rehabilitation protocol aims to promote healing, restore function, and minimize complications following surgery for patellar instability.

7. Primary Dislocation: Follow-Up

Follow-up may be scheduled 45 days after injury, with complete imaging screening: X-rays, MRI, or a CT scan. Regarding second-level imaging, MRI is generally recommended when ligamentous injury is suspected. On the other hand, when bony damage is suspected (with possible presence of osteochondral loose bodies), a CT scan is more appropriate [36]. On this occasion, the orthopedic surgeon will assess the effects of the conservative treatment and explain the risk factors for recurrence to the patient by identifying and quantifying the principal factors of instability and the PISS score. A return to sport is allowed three months after injury. In addition to the primary factors of instability, it is important for trauma surgeons to also focus on the so-called "secondary factors" of instability. These secondary factors encompass various aspects that can contribute to instability in the knee joint. One of these secondary factors is varus/valgus malalignment of the knee, which refers to the deviation of the knee joint from its normal alignment. This misalignment can place additional stress on the joint and contribute to instability. Another secondary factor is genu recurvatum, which is characterized by the hyperextension of the knee joint beyond its normal range. This excessive extension can compromise the stability of the knee and increase the risk of instability. Torsional malalignment of the lower extremities is also an important secondary factor to consider. This involves the abnormal rotation of the femur or tibia, such as increased femoral anteversion or increased internal torsion of the distal femur. These rotational abnormalities can affect the alignment and stability of the knee joint. Patellar dysplasia, classified by the Wiberg system [37], is another secondary factor that can contribute to instability. Patellar dysplasia refers to abnormal development or shape of the patella, which can affect its tracking and stability within the patellofemoral joint. Lastly, abnormal pronation of the subtalar joint can also be a secondary factor of instability. Excessive inward rolling of the foot during walking or running can impact the alignment and stability of the entire lower extremity, including the knee joint.

While the principal factors of instability must be detected via an accurate instrumental evaluation (MRI or CT scan), the secondary factors of instability can initially be assessed clinically. The physical examination starts by analyzing walking and standing positions, focusing on varus/valgus malalignment, torsional malalignment, and increased foot pronation. Any clinically evident torsional malalignment of the lower extremities, such as increased femoral anteversion or increased internal torsion of the distal femur, can be better defined via specific imaging evaluation (CT scan). Patellar dysplasia, classified via the Wiberg system, can be assessed on an axial view of radiographs of the patella. Abnormal pronation of the subtalar joint may require correction with orthotics. It is also suggested to examine the patient seated with their lower legs hanging. In many cases, when asked to actively extend the leg, a patient with patellar instability may present a so-called J sign, which means the patella moves resembling an inverted J while extending the knee. The apprehension test is positive in the majority of patients with patellar instability: the physician gently pushes the patella toward lateral at 0°–30°–60° and 90° of flexion with relaxed quadriceps. Avoidance or protective quadricep contraction indicates a positive test [38,39]

Patellar instability at 0°–30° of knee flexion reflects an insufficiency of passive stabilizers (mostly MPFL); instability at 0°–60° of knee flexion depends on an insufficiency of passive and often of static stabilizers (pathological TT-TG, trochlear dysplasia, patella alta, and valgus knee). Patellar instability at 0°–90° of knee flexion relies on complex rotational bony malalignment.

The study of the primary and secondary factors of instability gives us a complete framework of primary patellar instability. In the absence of osteochondral fractures, the treatment of primary patellar instability is usually conservative. If recurrence is highly probable (PISS $\geq$ 4) or important rotational malalignment is present, operative treatment should be considered. Considering the severity of the deformity, several surgical treatments can be taken into consideration. These include both arthroscopic and open MPFL repair or reconstruction, which have shown promising outcomes in recent studies [40–42]. Additionally, Fulkerson-type osteotomy has emerged as an effective approach in addressing complex cases [43]. Moreover, trochleoplasty has shown positive results in managing patellofemoral instability and can be considered a viable option for specific cases [43]. Lastly, the Goldthwait technique has also been explored as a potential treatment for patellofemoral instability and warrants consideration based on individual patient factors [44,45].

Understanding why the patient underwent primary patellar dislocation is a task for the orthopedic surgeon, allowing them to adopt the best therapeutic approach.

The prognosis of patellar instability can vary according to the disease course. After a first-time dislocation, nearly half of the subjects may experience further dislocations A history of chronic instability with recurrent dislocations may lead to progressive cartilage damage, thus potentially predisposing individuals to post-traumatic arthritis.

8. Conclusions

Patellofemoral instability can lead to different types of dislocations, making it necessary to establish an accurate diagnosis for primary patellar dislocation. The use of MRI is crucial to assess the extent of damage and determine the appropriate treatment options. Additionally, thorough post-treatment follow-up is essential, involving the analysis of both primary and secondary factors of instability. The orthopedic surgeon's role is to understand the underlying cause of the patient's primary patellar dislocation.

Author Contributions: Conceptualization, D.M.M. and R.G.; methodology, L.M.; validation, R.G.; investigation, C.M. and D.A.; resources, C.M. and D.A.; writing—original draft preparation, D.M.M. and R.G.; writing—review and editing, L.M. and G.M.P.; supervision, L.M. and G.M.P. All authors have read and agreed to the published version of the manuscript.

Funding: This research was funded by the Italian Ministry of Health, "Ricerca Corrente".

Institutional Review Board Statement: Not applicable.

Informed Consent Statement: Not applicable.

Data Availability Statement: The data presented in this study are available within the manuscript.

Conflicts of Interest: The authors declare no conflict of interest.

References

1. Arendt, E.A.; Dejour, D. Patella instability: Building bridges across the ocean a historic review. *Knee Surg. Sports Traumatol. Arthrosc.* **2013**, *21*, 279–293. [CrossRef]
2. Flandry, F.; Hommel, G. Normal anatomy and biomechanics of the knee. *Sports Med. Arthrosc. Rev.* **2011**, *19*, 82–92. [CrossRef] [PubMed]
3. Fox, A.J.S.; Wanivenhaus, F.; Rodeo, S.A. The basic science of the patella: Structure, composition, and function. *J. Knee Surg.* **2012**, *25*, 127–141. [CrossRef]
4. Van Kampen, A.; Huiskes, R. The three-dimensional tracking pattern of the human patella. *J. Orthop. Res.* **1990**, *8*, 372–382. [CrossRef] [PubMed]
5. Nagamine, R.; Otani, T.; White, S.E.; McCarthy, D.S.; Whiteside, L.A. Patellar tracking measurement in the normal knee. *J. Orthop. Res.* **1995**, *13*, 115–122. [CrossRef] [PubMed]
6. Wheatley, M.G.A.; Rainbow, M.J.; Clouthier, A.L. Patellofemoral Mechanics: A Review of Pathomechanics and Research Approaches. *Curr. Rev. Musculoskelet. Med.* **2020**, *13*, 326–337. [CrossRef]
7. Dejour, H.; Walch, G.; Nove-Josserand, L.; Guier, C. Factors of patellar instability: An anatomic radiographic study. *Knee Surg. Sports Traumatol. Arthrosc.* **1994**, *2*, 19–26. [CrossRef]

8. Crossley, K.M.; van Middelkoop, M.; Callaghan, M.J.; Collins, N.J.; Rathleff, M.S.; Barton, C.J. 2016 Patellofemoral pain consensus statement from the 4th International Patellofemoral Pain Research Retreat, Manchester. Part 2: Recommended physical interventions (exercise, taping, bracing, foot orthoses and combined interventions). *Br. J. Sports Med.* **2016**, *50*, 844–852. [CrossRef]
9. Dejour, D.; Saggin, P. The sulcus deepening trochleoplasty-the Lyon's procedure. *Int. Orthop.* **2010**, *34*, 311–316. [CrossRef]
10. Malghem, J.; Maldague, B. Patellofemoral joint: 30 degrees axial radiograph with lateral rotation of the leg. *Radiology* **1989**, *170*, 566–567. [CrossRef]
11. Caton, J. Method of measuring the height of the patella. *Acta Orthop. Belg.* **1989**, *55*, 385–386. [PubMed]
12. Lewallen, L.; McIntosh, A.; Dahm, D. First-Time Patellofemoral Dislocation: Risk Factors for Recurrent Instability. *J. Knee Surg.* **2015**, *28*, 303–309. [CrossRef] [PubMed]
13. Bayhan, I.A.; Kirat, A.; Alpay, Y.; Ozkul, B.; Kargin, D. Tibial tubercle-trochlear groove distance and angle are higher in children with patellar instability. *Knee Surg. Sports Traumatol. Arthrosc.* **2018**, *26*, 3566–3571. [CrossRef] [PubMed]
14. Polat, A.E.; Polat, B.; Gürpınar, T.; Sarı, E.; Çarkçı, E.; Erler, K. Tibial tubercle-trochlear groove (TT-TG) distance is a reliable measurement of increased rotational laxity in the knee with an anterior cruciate ligament injury. *Knee* **2020**, *27*, 1601–1607. [CrossRef]
15. Ahmad Khan, H.; Bashir Shah, A.; Kamal, Y. Vertical Patellar Dislocation: Reduction by the Push Up and Rotate Method, A Case Report and Literature Review. *Trauma. Mon.* **2016**, *21*, e24705. [CrossRef]
16. Udogwu, U.N.; Sabatini, C.S. Vertical patellar dislocation: A pediatric case report and review of the literature. *Orthop. Rev.* **2018**, *10*, 7688. [CrossRef]
17. Weber, A.E.; Nathani, A.; Dines, J.S.; Allen, A.A.; Shubin-Stein, B.E.; Arendt, E.A.; Bedi, A. An Algorithmic Approach to the Management of Recurrent Lateral Patellar Dislocation. *J. Bone Jt. Surg. Am.* **2016**, *98*, 417–427. [CrossRef]
18. Batra, S.; Arora, S. Habitual dislocation of patella: A review. *J. Clin. Orthop. Trauma.* **2014**, *5*, 245–251. [CrossRef]
19. Noda, M.; Saegusa, Y.; Kashiwagi, N.; Seto, Y. Surgical treatment for permanent dislocation of the patella in adults. *Orthopedics* **2011**, *34*, e948–e951. [CrossRef]
20. Fithian, D.C.; Paxton, E.W.; Stone, M.L.; Silva, P.; Davis, D.K.; Elias, D.A.; White, L.M. Epidemiology and natural history of acute patellar dislocation. *Am. J. Sports Med.* **2004**, *32*, 1114–1121. [CrossRef]
21. Pagliazzi, G.; Napoli, F.; Previtali, D.; Filardo, G.; Zaffagnini, S.; Candrian, C. A Meta-analysis of Surgical Versus Nonsurgical Treatment of Primary Patella Dislocation. *Arthroscopy* **2019**, *35*, 2469–2481. [CrossRef] [PubMed]
22. Kita, K.; Tanaka, Y.; Toritsuka, Y.; Amano, H.; Uchida, R.; Takao, R.; Horibe, S. Factors Affecting the Outcomes of Double-Bundle Medial Patellofemoral Ligament Reconstruction for Recurrent Patellar Dislocations Evaluated by Multivariate Analysis. *Am. J. Sports Med.* **2015**, *43*, 2988–2996. [CrossRef] [PubMed]
23. Frosch, K.-H.; Schmeling, A. A new classification system of patellar instability and patellar maltracking. *Arch. Orthop. Trauma. Surg.* **2016**, *136*, 485–497. [CrossRef] [PubMed]
24. Nikku, R.; Nietosvaara, Y.; Aalto, K.; Kallio, P.E. The mechanism of primary patellar dislocation: Trauma history of 126 patients. *Acta Orthop.* **2009**, *80*, 432–434. [CrossRef]
25. Placella, G.; Tei, M.M.; Sebastiani, E.; Criscenti, G.; Speziali, A.; Mazzola, C.; Georgoulis, A.; Cerulli, G. Shape and size of the medial patellofemoral ligament for the best surgical reconstruction: A human cadaveric study. *Knee Surg. Sports Traumatol. Arthrosc.* **2014**, *22*, 2327–2333. [CrossRef]
26. Sillanpää, P.J.; Peltola, E.; Mattila, V.M.; Kiuru, M.; Visuri, T.; Pihlajamäki, H. Femoral avulsion of the medial patellofemoral ligament after primary traumatic patellar dislocation predicts subsequent instability in men: A mean 7-year nonoperative follow-up study. *Am. J. Sports Med.* **2009**, *37*, 1513–1521. [CrossRef]
27. Elias, D.A.; White, L.M.; Fithian, D.C. Acute lateral patellar dislocation at MR imaging: Injury patterns of medial patellar soft-tissue restraints and osteochondral injuries of the inferomedial patella. *Radiology* **2002**, *225*, 736–743. [CrossRef]
28. Conlan, T.; Garth, W.P.; Lemons, J.E. Evaluation of the medial soft-tissue restraints of the extensor mechanism of the knee. *J. Bone Jt. Surg. Am.* **1993**, *75*, 682–693. [CrossRef]
29. McCrum, E.; Cooper, K.; Wittstein, J.; French, R.J. Imaging of Patellofemoral Instability. *Clin. Sports Med.* **2021**, *40*, 693–712. [CrossRef]
30. Maas, K.-J.; Warncke, M.L.; Leiderer, M.; Krause, M.; Dust, T.; Frings, J.; Frosch, K.-H.; Adam, G.; Henes, F.O.G. Diagnostic Imaging of Patellofemoral Instability. *ROFO Fortschr Geb Rontgenstr Nukl.* **2021**, *193*, 1019–1033. [CrossRef]
31. Arendt, E.A.; Askenberger, M.; Agel, J.; Tompkins, M.A. Risk of Redislocation After Primary Patellar Dislocation: A Clinical Prediction Model Based on Magnetic Resonance Imaging Variables. *Am. J. Sports Med.* **2018**, *46*, 3385–3390. [CrossRef] [PubMed]
32. Parikh, S.N.; Lykissas, M.G.; Gkiatas, I. Predicting Risk of Recurrent Patellar Dislocation. *Curr. Rev. Musculoskelet. Med.* **2018**, *11*, 253–260. [CrossRef] [PubMed]
33. Balcarek, P.; Oberthür, S.; Hopfensitz, S.; Frosch, S.; Walde, T.A.; Wachowski, M.M.; Schüttrumpf, J.P.; Stürmer, K.M. Which patellae are likely to redislocate? *Knee Surg. Sports Traumatol. Arthrosc.* **2014**, *22*, 2308–2314. [CrossRef]
34. Frings, J.; Balcarek, P.; Tscholl, P.; Liebensteiner, M.; Dirisamer, F.; Koenen, P. Conservative Versus Surgical Treatment for Primary Patellar Dislocation. *Dtsch. Arztebl. Int.* **2020**, *117*, 279–286. [CrossRef]
35. Medina Pérez, G.; Barrow, B.; Krueger, V.; Cruz, A.I. Treatment of Osteochondral Fractures After Acute Patellofemoral Instability: A Critical Analysis Review. *JBJS Rev.* **2022**, *10*, e21. [CrossRef]

36. Watts, R.E.; Gorbachova, T.; Fritz, R.C.; Saad, S.S.; Lutz, A.M.; Kim, J.; Chaudhari, A.S.; Shea, K.G.; Sherman, S.L.; Boutin, R.D Patellar Tracking: An Old Problem with New Insights. *Radiographics* **2023**, *43*, e220177. [CrossRef]
37. Panni, A.S.; Cerciello, S.; Maffulli, N.; Di Cesare, M.; Servien, E.; Neyret, P. Patellar shape can be a predisposing factor in patellar instability. *Knee Surg. Sports Traumatol. Arthrosc.* **2011**, *19*, 663–670. [CrossRef]
38. Hughston, J.C. Subluxation of the patella. *J. Bone Jt. Surg. Am.* **1968**, *50*, 1003–1026. [CrossRef]
39. Fairbank, H.A. Internal Derangement of the Knee in Children and Adolescents: (Section of Orthopaedics). *Proc. R. Soc. Med.* **1937**, *30*, 427–432.
40. Alshaban, R.M.; Ghaddaf, A.A.; Alghamdi, D.M.; Aghashami, A.; Alqrni, A.; Alyasi, A.A.; Bogari, H.; Qadi, S. Operative versus non-operative management of primary patellar dislocation: A systematic review and network meta-analysis. *Injury* **2023**, *54*, 110926. [CrossRef]
41. Xu, T.; Xu, L.-H.; Li, X.-Z.; Fu, H.-J.; Zhou, Y. Original surgical technique for the treatment of patellofemoral instability after failure of conservative treatment. *Orthop. Traumatol. Surg. Res.* **2023**, 103657. [CrossRef]
42. Herdea, A.; Pencea, V.; Lungu, C.N.; Charkaoui, A.; Ulici, A. A Prospective Cohort Study on Quality of Life among the Pediatric Population after Surgery for Recurrent Patellar Dislocation. *Child* **2021**, *8*, 830. [CrossRef] [PubMed]
43. Wolfe, S.; Varacallo, M.; Thomas, J.D.; Carroll, J.J.; Kahwaji, C.I. Patellar Instability. In *StatPearls*; StatPearls Publishing: Treasure Island, FL, USA, 2023.
44. Trivellas, M.; Arshi, A.; Beck, J.J. Roux-Goldthwait and Medial Patellofemoral Ligament Reconstruction for Patella Realignment in the Skeletally Immature Patient. *Arthrosc. Tech.* **2019**, *8*, e1479–e1483. [CrossRef] [PubMed]
45. Felli, L.; Capello, A.G.; Lovisolo, S.; Chiarlone, F.; Alessio-Mazzola, M. Goldthwait technique for patellar instability: Surgery of the past or here to stay procedure? A systematic review of the literature. *Musculoskelet. Surg.* **2019**, *103*, 107–113. [CrossRef] [PubMed]

Disclaimer/Publisher's Note: The statements, opinions and data contained in all publications are solely those of the individual author(s) and contributor(s) and not of MDPI and/or the editor(s). MDPI and/or the editor(s) disclaim responsibility for any injury to people or property resulting from any ideas, methods, instructions or products referred to in the content.

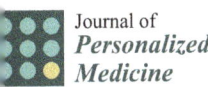

Study Protocol

A Longitudinal Analysis of the Internal Rotation and Shift (IRO/Shift) Test Following Arthroscopic Repair of Superior Rotator Cuff Lesions

René Schwesig [1], George Fieseler [2], Jakob Cornelius [1,2], Julia Sendler [1,2], Stephan Schulze [1], Souhail Hermassi [3], Karl-Stefan Delank [1] and Kevin Laudner [4,*]

1 Department of Orthopedic and Trauma Surgery, Martin-Luther-University Halle-Wittenberg, 06120 Halle, Germany
2 Clinic for Orthopedic and Trauma Surgery, Sports Medicine, Clinic Hannoversch Münden, 34346 Hannoversch Münden, Germany
3 Physical Education Department, College of Education, Qatar University, Doha 2713, Qatar
4 Department of Health Sciences, University of Colorado Colorado Springs, Colorado Springs, CO 80918, USA
* Correspondence: klaudner@uccs.edu

Abstract: Although the use of clinical tests to diagnose superior rotator cuff pathology is common, there is paucity in the research regarding the accuracy of such tests following arthroscopic repair. The aim of this study was to determine the accuracy of the IRO/Shift test compared to the Jobe test at 3 months and 6 months post-surgery for superior rotator cuff repair. Arthroscopic repair was conducted on 51 patients who were subsequently seen for clinical evaluation at 3 and 6 months following surgery. At 3 months post-surgery only 27% of the patients had a negative IRO/Shift test and 18% had a negative Jobe test. However, at 6 months 88% of the patients presented with a negative IRO/Shift test and 61% a negative Jobe test. When compared to each other, the IRO/Shift test and the Jobe test had 90% agreement pre-operatively, 71% agreement at 3 months post-surgery, and 67% agreement at 6 months. These results demonstrate that the accuracy of the IRO/Shift test and the Jobe test improved between 3 and 6 months following arthroscopic surgery of the superior rotator cuff, with the IRO/Shift test having better accuracy.

Keywords: arthroscopic surgery; clinical test; diagnostic accuracy; shoulder; supraspinatus

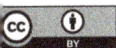

1. Introduction

The accurate diagnosis of superior rotator cuff lesions is a challenging process. Clinicians often use a combination of techniques including various special tests such as the Jobe test, shoulder shrug sign, full can test, shoulder drop arm test, and others, as well as advanced imaging to maximize their clinical impression [1]. Unfortunately, there is still some degree of error that comes with these clinical tests, with some tests reporting strong sensitivity, but poor specificity or vice versa [2–5]. Previous research has also investigated the use of predictive models, which combine various special tests for increased accuracy [3,4]. This has led to many reports stressing the importance of using multiple tests to increase diagnostic accuracy, rather than relying on one test [2,6–8]. As such, clinicians are continuously trying to stay innovative in what procedures they use during their clinical examinations, which will allow them to better isolate the desired soft tissue structure, or structures, such as the supraspinatus tendon and therefore, increase the accuracy of their diagnoses. Furthermore, the recurrent application of clinical tests following surgery and rehabilitation is useful to supervise the process of convalescence. The conversion of a pathological clinical test to negative results over time demonstrates the appropriate recovery of a torn and surgically repaired tendon.

One of the more recent tests developed for the assessment of superior rotator cuff pathology, the internal rotation and shift test (IRO/Shift test), was originally described by

Fieseler et al. [9]. This test has been shown to be both a reliable and valid technique for identifying superior rotator cuff lesions [9–11]. More specifically, these authors reported an intrarater reliability of ICC = 0.73 and an interrater reliability of ICC = 0.89, as well as 92% sensitivity, 67% specificity, 86% positive predictive value, and 80% negative predictive value. Subsequent research also found that the IRO/Shift test was comparable to the Jobe test [12], which has been viewed as the gold standard of testing for these types of lesions [2,5]. This study reported the IRO/Shift test to have 96% sensitivity, 50% specificity, 73% positive predictive value, 91% negative predictive value, and an accuracy of 77%, while the Jobe test had 89% sensitivity, 60% specificity, 76% positive predictive value, 80% negative predictive value, and an accuracy of 77%. Although this previous work has demonstrated that the IRO/Shift test is an accurate and valid tool in the diagnosis of this pathology, there is paucity in the research regarding the outcomes of using this technique among post-operative patients. Understanding the usefulness of this special test throughout the post-surgical rehabilitation process could be a critical tool for physicians and physiotherapists as they attempt to accurately assess the healing of the tendon and its correlation with the physical demands of the rehabilitation process. Therefore, the purpose of the current study was to determine how long following the arthroscopic repair of a superior rotator cuff lesion would patients present with a positive IRO/Shift test. More specifically, this study examined the accuracy of using the IRO/Shift test compared to the Jobe test at 3 months and 6 months post-surgery for superior rotator cuff repair.

2. Materials and Methods

2.1. Subjects

Eighty-seven subjects (51 male, 36 female) volunteered to participate in this study (age: 53.6 ± 12.5 years; height: 1.76 ± 0.09 m; weight: 83.0 ± 15.3 kg, BMI: 26.7 ± 3.51 kg/m^2). All subjects were 18 years of age or older (age range: 20.9–74.7 years) and presented with a radiologically confirmed structural lesion of the superior rotator cuff, pain, and persistent malfunction of the glenohumeral joint. Prior to their introduction to this study, all subjects had completed a conservative rehabilitation program prescribed by their general physician, conducted under the supervision of a physiotherapist, which resulted in no reduction in their shoulder symptoms. During or after this conservative treatment, magnetic resonance imaging (MRI) was then determined to be necessary to detect the extent of structural pathology and the reasoning for their lack of improvement. Upon review of the MRIs, by an experienced radiologist, structural lesions of the supraspinatus were identified. Following the MRI, all patients were then referred to a single shoulder unit for specialized examination and to determine if surgical intervention was indicated.

Exclusion criteria included a restricted shoulder range of motion, non-traumatic glenohumeral instability, fracture/osseous pathology, acute dislocation, glenohumeral arthrosis, or arthritis. Prior to any data collection, all subjects provided consent as approved by the ethical committee of Martin-Luther-University Halle-Wittenberg (approval number: 2018-05). In total, 59% (51/87) of the patients presented with a radiologically diagnosed superior rotator cuff lesion pre-operatively, which was confirmed intra-operatively. Arthroscopic repair was then conducted on these 51 patients. All surgeries were exclusively performed by an experienced orthopedic shoulder surgeon with more than 20 years of shoulder surgery experience and who performs more than 200 arthroscopic or open surgical procedures per year.

2.2. Procedures

This research study used a prospective, blinded study design (Figure 1).

During the initial (pre-operative) clinical examination, two examiners (a surgeon and a resident) performed both the IRO/Shift test and the Jobe test to determine the integrity of the superior rotator cuff tendon. Following arthroscopic repair, each subject returned to the resident who performed the same clinical examinations in the 3-month and 6-month post-operative time periods. During the 3- and 6-month examinations, the resident was blinded to the patient's status, meaning the resident was unaware of their surgical status.

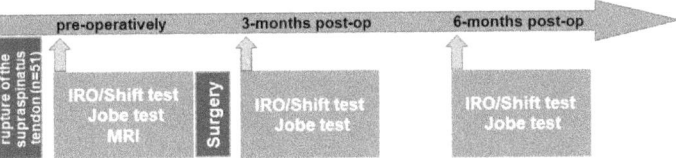

Figure 1. Prospective, blinded study design.

The IRO/Shift test was performed in accordance with Fieseler et al. [9]. For this test, patients stood in a relaxed position and actively moved their involved shoulder into internal rotation and adduction, by rotating the arm behind their back and then sliding their hand superiorly along their spine, attempting to reach the highest or most superior vertebral spinous process. At their end range of active motion, the clinician then provided a subsequent passive movement of their shoulder into further internal rotation and adduction (i.e., moving the arm and hand more superiorly up the spine) until the end range of passive motion. If increased pain and avoidance was present during this end range of passive motion, the test was considered positive. However, the clinician then needed to rule out possible involvement of the long head of the biceps tendon. If the long head of the biceps tendon was found to be involved (e.g., a positive O'Brien test), then the IRO/Shift test was considered negative for superior rotator cuff pathology. If the long head of the biceps tendon was not found to be involved, then the IRO/Shift test was considered positive.

2.3. Statistical Analysis

All statistical analyses were conducted using SPSS version 28.0 for Windows (IBM, Armonk, NY, USA). Arthroscopic findings were used as the gold standard to calculate the sensitivity and specificity (95% confidence interval) of both the IRO/Shift test and the Jobe test. The percentage of positive tests at pre-operation, and 3 and 6 months post-surgery were calculated and reported for both the IRO/Shift test and the Jobe test. The accuracy of the IRO/Shift test was compared to the Jobe test using a Chi-squared analysis. The observed accuracy (percentage) of both tests was defined as consistent negative and positive results and assessed using a four-field table. In this context, a Chi-squared analysis was used to determine the relationship between positive and negative findings for each test in order to illustrate the recovery process.

3. Results

The sensitivity of the IRO/Shift test (92%) and the Jobe test (94%) among the 87 patients who initially received a clinical examination prior to any surgical intervention was comparable with each other (Table 1). With respect to specificity, prior to shoulder surgery, a difference of 10% (IRO/Shift test: 68% vs. Jobe test: 78%) was calculated when confirmed with MRI findings.

Table 1. IRO/Shift and Jobe test performance prior to shoulder surgery (confirmed with MRI).

Test	Sensitivity (95% CI)	Specificity (95% CI)
IRO/Shift (%)	92 (87–100)	68 (51–85)
Jobe (%)	94 (88–100)	78 (64–91)

IRO/Shift: internal rotation and shift; CI: confidence interval.

Among the 51 patients who underwent rotator cuff repair, 22 had a single row repair, 16 had a double row repair, and 13 had debridement only. Figure 2 displays the number of positive IRO/Shift tests longitudinally based on surgical procedure.

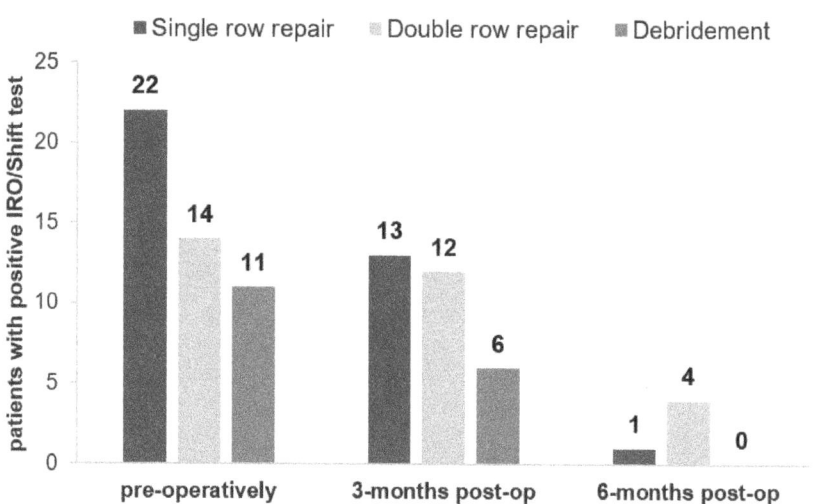

Figure 2. Number of positive IRO/Shift tests longitudinally based on surgical procedure ($n = 51$).

Among the 36 patients who underwent arthroscopic surgery, but did not have a rotator cuff tear, 15 had a positive IRO/Shift test and 8 had a positive Jobe test pre-surgery. At 3 months post-surgery there were six positive IRO/Shift and six positive Jobe tests, while at 6 months there was only one positive IRO/Shift and two positive Jobe tests.

In total, 47 of the 51 surgical patients presented with a positive IRO/Shift test pre-surgery, while 48 presented with a positive Jobe test (Figure 3). At 3 months post-surgery there were 31 positive IRO/Shift tests and 36 positive Jobe tests. Meaning only 39% (20/51) had a negative IRO/Shift test and 29% (15/51) had a negative Jobe test at 3 months post-surgery. However, at 6 months post-surgery there were only 5 remaining positive IRO/Shift tests and 18 positive Jobe tests. This resulted in 90% of the patients (46/51) presenting with a negative IRO/Shift test and 65% (33/51) of the patients presenting with a negative Jobe test at 6 months post-surgery. When compared to each other over time, the observed accuracy between the tests decreased. The IRO/Shift test and Jobe test had 90% agreement (i.e., accuracy) pre-operatively, 71% agreement at 3 months post-surgery, and 67% agreement at 6 months (Table 2).

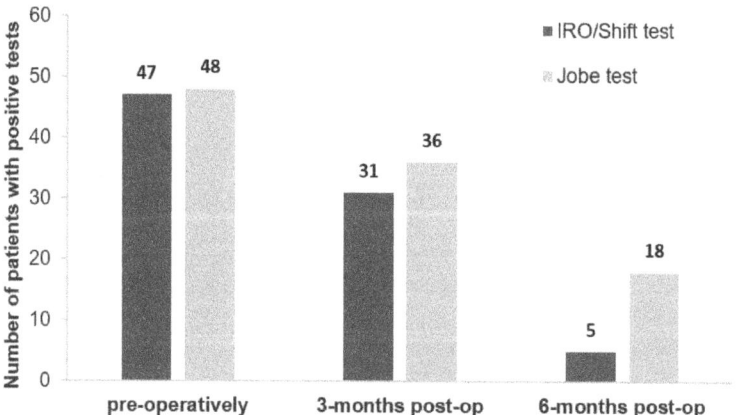

Figure 3. Number of positive IRO/Shift tests and Jobe tests longitudinally. Patients ($n = 51$) with arthroscopically confirmed superior rotator cuff lesions.

Table 2. Observed accuracy (Jobe vs. IRO/Shift) depending on examination points for the injured sample ($n = 51$).

Time Point	Observed Accuracy			Chi-Squared Test (p-Value)
	Negative (n)	Positive (n)	%	
Pre-operative	1	45	90	2.87 (0.091)
3 months post-op	10	26	71	**6.72 (0.010)**
6 months post-op	31	3	67	1.48 (0.224)

IRO/Shift: internal rotation and shift; post-op: post-operative. Significant relationship is bolded.

The only statistically significant finding was at 3 months post-surgery (Chi-Squared: 6.72, $p = 0.010$). In relation to the healing process, the number of negative matched findings increased sharply from $n = 1$ (pre-surgery) to $n = 10$ (3-months post-surgery) and $n = 31$ (6 months post-surgery). Conversely, the number of concurrent positive findings decreased from $n = 45$ to $n = 26$ and $n = 3$ during this observation period (Table 2).

4. Discussion

The IRO/Shift test has been shown to be a reliable and valid technique for assessing the presence of superior rotator cuff pathology. However, no research has investigated the use of this special test following arthroscopic rotator cuff repair alongside using a longitudinal approach to guide the rehabilitation process and tendon recovery. The results of this study are the first to compare the use of the IRO/Shift test and the Jobe test at 3 months and 6 months post-surgery. These results demonstrate that patients with superior rotator cuff repair present with progressively negative IRO/Shift test and Jobe test findings between 3 and 6 months post-surgery.

Following arthroscopic repair, rotator cuff tendons need a substantial amount of time to heal, with most retears occurring between 6 and 26 weeks (primarily between 12 and 26 weeks) following surgical repair [13]. At 3 months post-surgery, 61% of the patients in the current study still had a positive IRO/Shift test, while 71% still had a positive Jobe test. By 6 months, those positive tests fell to only 10% for the IRO/Shift test and 35% for the Jobe test. This may be explained by the timing of tendon repair and regeneration during the healing process, as well as different forces exerted between the two clinical tests. The Jobe test emphasizes a lever load testing strength via an extended arm placing traction on the tendon, while the IRO/Shift test places a tensile load on the tendon without leverage. Voleti et al. [14] noted that tendon stiffness and collagen reorganization continue to increase from 2 to 16 weeks post-surgery in rats with supraspinatus repair. These authors also reported that less than 10% of the supraspinatus recapitalizes compared to the non-injured limb at 12 weeks post-surgery. Some research has shown that this remodeling phase, where the collagen aligns with stress/strain, predominantly occurs from 1 to 2 months post injury/surgery and can continue for more than 12 months [15]. This may also help explain why the IRO/Shift test, which applies tensile stress to the tendon, had slightly better accuracy following surgery than the Jobe test, which assesses the contractile strength of the muscle.

The differences in stress placed on the rotator cuff tendons by the IRO/Shift and the Jobe tests may potentially explain the divergent correlations of the two tests' accuracy related to the time of examination throughout the pathological process (pre- and post-operatively) (Table 2). From a statistical point of view, the observed accuracy between both tests steadily decreased from 90% (pre-operatively) to 71% (3 months post-operatively) and 67% (6 months post-operatively). The only statistically significant relationship was found during the second examination (3 months post-surgery) (Chi-squared: 6.72; $p = 0.010$). From a biological and orthopedic perspective, this relationship in the 3-month post-surgery period may have occurred due to the biological demand placed on the tendon while it was still healing. Conversely, during the 6-month examination, the difference in tissue loads between tests may have been more prominent because of the surgically fixed tendon to the footprint and the ability to resist tensile force produced by the IRO/Shift test, and the lack of contractile muscle strength generated by an active movement of the arm during the Jobe test. These findings also support Young's modulus of elasticity, which notes that following injury collagen is largely disorganized and has a lower resistance to tension and compression. However, throughout the remodeling phase, elasticity continually increases to roughly 80% of the contralateral tendon, while the cross-sectional area and viscoelastic phase angle (tensile strength) are 3 and 1.5 times greater, respectively [16].

In accordance with tendon healing, previous research has shown that multiple functional characteristics significantly improve between 3 and 6 months following arthroscopic rotator cuff repair. For example, He et al. [17] investigated the clinical outcomes of 89 patients who underwent arthroscopic rotator cuff repair using the Southern California Orthopedic Institute row method and found that visual analog scale scores, University of California Los Angeles (UCLA) scores, and Constant–Murley scores, as well as abduction and forward flexion range of motion were all better at 6 months compared to 3 months. Similarly, other research has demonstrated that most improvements in shoulder range of motion (flexion and external rotation), pain, and function occurred by 6 months post-surgery [18,19]. The results of the current study support these previous findings and provide further insight into the use of clinical testing following arthroscopic repair.

In contrast to the IRO/Shift test, which stresses tension on the superior rotator cuff, the Jobe test emphasizes muscle contractile strength to keep the shoulder in a position of internal rotation and elevation. As such, the authors of this study hypothesized that the most of the patients would present with a negative Jobe test 6 months following surgery. This was based on previous studies which have shown increases in muscular strength around the 6-month post-surgery period [19,20]. Unfortunately, only 65% (31/51) of the patients presented with a negative Jobe test at 6 months post-surgery, compared to 90% of the patients with a negative IRO/Shift test. This suggests that test conversion of the IRO/Shift may allow for a quicker return to negative findings following arthroscopic repair due to the stretch and tensile load placed on the tendon compared to the Jobe test. Regardless, clinicians should be discouraged from relying on only one test for diagnosis [2,6–8]; therefore, the authors of this study recommend the use of both tests for pre-operative diagnosis and as a tool for post-operative follow-up during rehabilitation and tendon healing.

There are a few limitations of this study worth noting. First, the research participants were relatively young (age: 54 ± 13 years, 33% of patients were younger than 50 years). Previous research has shown that post-operative outcomes can decrease as age increases [21]. Therefore, care should be taken when interpreting these results among older patients. Next, this study identified that negative findings improved for both the IRO/Shift and the Jobe test between 3 and 6 months post-surgery but did not specify an exact time period over this 3-month period. Similarly, the results of this study looked at the short-term outcomes using these clinical tests. Future research should investigate the accuracy of these tests during longer intervals (e.g., 9 months, 12 months, and 24 months post-surgery). Similarly, future research should investigate if patients who still present with a positive IRO/Shift test at the end of the follow-up period (24 months) demonstrate a recurrence of tears or lack of reparative fusion on reimaging. Tendon healing was not monitored post-operatively, so it is impossible to conclude if all tendons were healing at a similar pace. However, all patients that presented with a negative IRO/Shift or Jobe test reported pain-free shoulders with good range of motion and function during daily activities.

5. Conclusions

The observed accuracy of the IRO/Shift test and the Jobe test decreased during the observational period (pre-surgery, 3 months post-arthroscopic surgery, and 6 months post-arthroscopic surgery of the superior rotator cuff), depending on the different requirements of the tests and the healing process. This may be due to better alignment of the tensile load accumulated during the IRO/Shift test throughout the healing process. Regardless, both tests demonstrated a high level of sensitivity and specificity. Therefore, these tests should be considered in the post-operative evaluation of superior rotator cuff pathology and during the rehabilitation process.

Author Contributions: Conceptualization, G.F., R.S., J.S., J.C., S.H. and K.L.; methodology, G.F., R.S., J.S., J.C., S.S., S.H., K.-S.D. and K.L.; software, G.F., R.S., J.S., J.C., S.S., S.H., K.-S.D. and K.L.; validation, G.F., R.S., J.S., J.C., S.S., K.-S.D. and K.L.; formal analysis, G.F., R.S., J.S., J.C., S.S., S.H. and K.L.; investigation, G.F., R.S., J.S., J.C. and K.L.; resources, G.F., R.S., J.S., J.C., K.-S.D. and K.L.; data curation, G.F., R.S., J.S., J.C., S.H. and K.L.; writing original draft preparation, G.F., R.S., J.S., J.C., S.S., K.-S.D. and K.L.; writing review and editing, G.F., R.S., J.S., J.C., S.H., K.-S.D. and K.L.; visualization, G.F., R.S., J.S., J.C., S.S., S.H. and K.L.; supervision, G.F., R.S., J.S., J.C., S.S., S.H., K.-S.D. and K.L.; project administration, G.F., R.S. and K.L. All authors have read and agreed to the published version of the manuscript.

Funding: This research received no external funding.

Institutional Review Board Statement: This study was approved by the Ethics Commission of the Martin-Luther-University Halle-Wittenberg (reference number: 2018-05).

Informed Consent Statement: All subjects provided informed consent.

Data Availability Statement: Please contact the corresponding author for inquiries regarding study data.

Conflicts of Interest: The authors declare no conflict of interest.

References

1. Hawkins, R.J.; Bokor, D.J. *Clinical Evaluation of Shoulder Problems. The Shoulder*; Saunders: Philadelphia, PA, USA, 1990.
2. Lädermann, A.; Meynard, T.; Denard, P.J.; Ibrahim, M.; Saffarini, M.; Collin, P. Reliable diagnosis of posterosuperior rotator cuff tears requires a combination of clinical tests. *Knee Surg. Sports Traumatol. Arthrosc.* **2021**, *29*, 2118–2133. [CrossRef] [PubMed]
3. van Kampen, D.A.; van den Berg, T.; van der Woude, H.J.; Castelein, R.M.; Scholtes, V.A.; Terwee, C.B.; Willems, W.J. The diagnostic value of the combination of patient characteristics, history, and clinical shoulder tests for the diagnosis of rotator cuff tear. *J. Orthop. Surg. Res.* **2014**, *9*, 70. [CrossRef] [PubMed]
4. Águila-Ledesma, I.R.; Córdova-Fonseca, J.L.; Medina-Pontaza, O.; A Núñez-Gómez, D.; Calvache-García, C.; Pérez-Atanasio, J.M.; Torres-González, R. Diagnostic value of a predictive model for complete ruptures of the rotator cuff associated to subacromial impingement. *Acta Ortop. Mex.* **2017**, *31*, 108–112. [PubMed]
5. Jain, N.B.; Luz, J.; Higgins, L.D.; Dong, Y.; Warner, J.J.P.; Matzkin, E.; Katz, J.N. The Diagnostic Accuracy of Special Tests for Rotator Cuff Tear: The ROW Cohort Study. *Am. J. Phys. Med. Rehabil.* **2017**, *96*, 176–183. [CrossRef] [PubMed]
6. Cadogan, A.; McNair, P.J.; Laslett, M.; Hing, W.A. Diagnostic Accuracy of Clinical Examination and Imaging Findings for Identifying Subacromial Pain. *PLoS ONE* **2016**, *11*, e0167738. [CrossRef] [PubMed]
7. Sgroi, M.; Loitsch, T.; Reichel, H.; Kappe, T. Diagnostic Value of Clinical Tests for Supraspinatus Tendon Tears. *Arthrosc. J. Arthrosc. Relat. Surg.* **2018**, *34*, 2326–2333. [CrossRef]
8. Somerville, L.E.; Willits, K.; Johnson, A.M.; Litchfield, R.; Lebel, M.-E.; Moro, J.; Bryant, D. Clinical Assessment of Physical Examination Maneuvers for Rotator Cuff Lesions. *Am. J. Sports Med.* **2014**, *42*, 1911–1919. [CrossRef]
9. Fieseler, G.; Laudner, K.; Sendler, J.; Cornelius, J.; Schulze, S.; Lehmann, W.; Hermassi, S.; Delank, K.-S.; Schwesig, R. The internal rotation and shift-test for the detection of superior lesions of the rotator cuff: Reliability and clinical performance. *JSES Int.* **2022**, *6*, 495–499. [CrossRef]
10. Fieseler, G. Der IRO-/Shift-Test zur klinischen Diagnostik superiorer Rotatorenmanschettendefekte. *Arthroskopie* **2021**, *34*, 456–458. [CrossRef]
11. Fieseler, G.; Sendler, J.; Cornelius, J.; Schulze, S.; Delank, K.S.; Bartels, T.; Schwesig, R. Der Innenrotations/Shift-Test; Erweiterung der manuellen Diagnostik bei superioren Rotatorenmanschettendefekten—Übereinstimmung der klinischen Untersuchung mit fachradiologischen MRT-Befunden. *Sport. Orthop. Traumatol.* **2020**, *32*, 192–193. [CrossRef]
12. Fieseler, G.; Schwesig, R.; Sendler, J.; Cornelius, J.; Schulze, S.; Lehmann, W.; Hermassi, S.; Delank, K.-S.; Laudner, K. IRO/Shift Test Is Comparable to the Jobe Test for Detection of Supraspinatus Lesions. *J. Pers. Med.* **2022**, *12*, 1422. [CrossRef] [PubMed]
13. Iannotti, J.P.; Deutsch, A.; Green, A.; Rudicel, S.; Christensen, J.; Marraffino, S.; Rodeo, S. Time to failure after rotator cuff repair: A prospective imaging study. *J. Bone Jt. Surg. Am.* **2013**, *95*, 965–971. [CrossRef] [PubMed]
14. Voleti, P.B.; Buckley, M.R.; Soslowsky, L.J. Tendon Healing: Repair and Regeneration. *Annu. Rev. Biomed. Eng.* **2012**, *14*, 47–71. [CrossRef] [PubMed]
15. Leadbetter, W.B. Cell-Matrix Response in Tendon Injury. *Clin. Sports Med.* **1992**, *11*, 533–578. [CrossRef] [PubMed]
16. Nagasawa, K.; Noguchi, M.; Ikoma, K.; Kubo, T. Static and dynamic biomechanical properties of the regenerating rabbit Achilles tendon. *Clin. Biomech.* **2008**, *23*, 832–838. [CrossRef] [PubMed]

17. He, H.B.; Wang, T.; Wang, M.C.; Zhu, H.F.; Meng, Y.; Pan, C.L.; Hu, Y.; Chao, X.M.; Yang, C.Y.; Wang, M. Tendon-to-bone healing after repairing full-thickness rotator cuff tear with a triple-loaded single-row method in young patients. *BMC Musculoskelet. Disord.* **2021**, *22*, 305. [CrossRef] [PubMed]
18. Baysal, D.; Balyk, R.; Otto, D.; Luciak-Corea, C.; Beaupre, L. Functional Outcome and Health-Related Quality of Life after Surgical Repair of Full-Thickness Rotator Cuff Tear Using a Mini-Open Technique. *Am. J. Sports Med.* **2005**, *33*, 1346–1355. [CrossRef] [PubMed]
19. Charousset, C.; Grimberg, J.; Duranthon, L.D.; Bellaïche, L.; Petrover, D.; Kalra, K. The Time for Functional Recovery After Arthroscopic Rotator Cuff Repair: Correlation With Tendon Healing Controlled by Computed Tomography Arthrography. *Arthrosc. J. Arthrosc. Relat. Surg.* **2008**, *24*, 25–33. [CrossRef] [PubMed]
20. Rokito, A.S.; Zuckerman, J.D.; Gallagher, M.A.; Cuomo, F. Strength after surgical repair of the rotator cuff. *J. Shoulder Elb. Surg.* **1996**, *5*, 12–17. [CrossRef] [PubMed]
21. Tashjian, R.Z.; Hollins, A.M.; Kim, H.-M.; Teefey, S.A.; Middleton, W.D.; Steger-May, K.; Galatz, L.M.; Yamaguchi, K. Factors Affecting Healing Rates after Arthroscopic Double-Row Rotator Cuff Repair. *Am. J. Sports Med.* **2010**, *38*, 2435–2442. [CrossRef] [PubMed]

MDPI
St. Alban-Anlage 66
4052 Basel
Switzerland
www.mdpi.com

Journal of Personalized Medicine Editorial Office
E-mail: jpm@mdpi.com
www.mdpi.com/journal/jpm

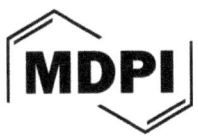

Disclaimer/Publisher's Note: The statements, opinions and data contained in all publications are solely those of the individual author(s) and contributor(s) and not of MDPI and/or the editor(s). MDPI and/or the editor(s) disclaim responsibility for any injury to people or property resulting from any ideas, methods, instructions or products referred to in the content.